ADDICTED
to Opioids

Jennifer Skancke

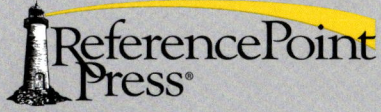

San Diego, CA

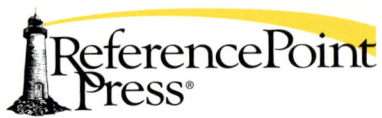

© 2020 ReferencePoint Press, Inc.
Printed in the United States

For more information, contact:
ReferencePoint Press, Inc.
PO Box 27779
San Diego, CA 92198
www.ReferencePointPress.com

ALL RIGHTS RESERVED.
No part of this work covered by the copyright hereon may be reproduced or used in any form or by any means—graphic, electronic, or mechanical, including photocopying, recording, taping, web distribution, or information storage retrieval systems—without the written permission of the publisher.

LIBRARY OF CONGRESS CATALOGING-IN-PUBLICATION DATA

Name: Skancke, Jennifer, author.
Title: Addicted to Opioids/by Jennifer Skancke.
Description: San Diego, CA: ReferencePoint Press, Inc., 2020. | Series:
  Addicted | Audience: Grade 9 to 12. | Includes bibliographical references
  and index.
Identifiers: LCCN 2019016233 (print) | LCCN 2019017880 (ebook) | ISBN
  9781682825723 (eBook) | ISBN 9781682825716 (hardback)
Subjects: LCSH: Opioid abuse—Juvenile literature. | Opioid
  abuse—Treatment—Juvenile literature.
Classification: LCC RC568.O45 (ebook) | LCC RC568.O45 S53 2020 (print) | DDC
  362.29—dc23
LC record available at https://lccn.loc.gov/2019016233

Contents

Introduction   4
The Opioid Crisis: A Public Health Emergency

Chapter One   9
The Scope of Opioid Addiction

Chapter Two   20
What Influences Opioid Addiction?

Chapter Three   30
How People Become Addicted to Opioids

Chapter Four   40
Living with Opioid Addiction

Chapter Five   52
Overcoming Opioid Addiction

Source Notes   64
Get Help and Information   67
For Further Research   70
Index   72
Picture Credits   79
About the Author   80

Introduction

The Opioid Crisis: A Public Health Emergency

Cortney was sixteen years old when she tried a prescription opioid for the first time. It was a decision that would change the course of her life. She says:

> My first prescription opioid pill came from a girlfriend, who told me that it was safe and harmless because it came from her doctor. But that pill flipped a switch inside me that took away my emotional pain and made me numb. I knew hard drugs were illegal and taboo, but I didn't think that *these* pills were dangerous. I had no idea that I could actually get addicted—I just knew that I felt sick when I stopped taking them. I went from being an honors student and varsity athlete, to a high school dropout in just one year. I tried to go to college after getting my GED, but my life revolved around using pills. I was so dependent on the pills, that I became a shell of the person that I used to be.[1]

Cortney spent the next three years of her life in full-blown addiction. After a failed intentional overdose at age nineteen, she decided to face her addiction. With the help of recovery resources, supportive peers, and dedicated counselors, she stopped using opioids and has been in recovery for over ten years.

Cortney was like one of the estimated 2.1 million Americans who battled an addiction to opioids in 2017, according to the Substance Abuse and Mental Health Services Administration. Opioids are a class of drugs that includes pain medications such as oxycodone, hydrocodone, codeine, and morphine and that are available legally by prescription, as well as the illegal street drug heroin and synthetic opioids like fentanyl and its analogues (fentanyl-related substances). These drugs not only provide relief from pain but also produce a euphoric feeling that is highly addictive—which also makes them very deadly. According to the Centers for Disease Control and Prevention (CDC), from 1999 to 2017, nearly four hundred thousand Americans died from an opioid overdose, leading health officials to declare the high mortality rate an epidemic.

> "I had no idea that I could actually get addicted."[1]
>
> —Cortney, a former opioid user

The Rise of the Opioid Epidemic

The current epidemic began in the 1990s, when medical organizations and pain specialists argued that pain was going untreated in the United States. They advocated for the medical community to pay more attention to pain management. However, many doctors had limited training in evaluating and treating both chronic and acute pain, especially noncancer pain or pain associated with surgeries. Around the same time, pharmaceutical companies, having developed new pain medications, heavily marketed these drugs to doctors. They touted them as being safe and less addictive than morphine, a highly addictive opiate previously used to treat pain. Drug representatives provided doctors with free samples as well as gifts and offers for all-expense-paid trips to medical symposiums. These marketing efforts, along with pressure from the medical community to eliminate patients' pain, led doctors to prescribe opioid painkillers at much higher rates than they had previously.

Because of no clear consensus on dosage levels, however, doctors did not prescribe opioids in consistent ways—either for the right usage or in doses that protected patients from developing a dependency on the drugs. Painkillers became a routine treatment for all kinds of chronic conditions, from back pain to osteoarthritis and chronic, painful diseases like fibromyalgia. As doctors wrote more prescriptions (with a peak of 282 million prescriptions filled in 2012), more patients became dependent on opioids.

This dependency led some patients to misuse their prescriptions. Some got addicted, while some sold the drugs to others who misused them. According to the CDC, the rise in the number of opioid prescriptions correlates to the increase in the number of opioid overdose deaths. In fact, 218,000 Americans died from prescription opioid overdoses from 1999 to 2017, with the rate of deaths five times higher in 2017 than in 1999. Neither doctors nor patients knew just how addictive opioids would be.

Fentanyl, a synthetic opioid pain reliever used to treat severe pain, is thirty to fifty times more potent than heroin. It recently surpassed heroin as the leading cause of opioid overdose deaths.

However, some doctors, sensing a problem was underway, sought to limit or better control opioid use in their patients by writing fewer prescriptions. Drug dealers took advantage of the fact that it was becoming harder to get opioid prescriptions by flooding the streets with inexpensive heroin, an extremely strong and illegal opioid that leads to quick highs. Heroin attracted opioid users who no longer had access to prescription painkillers or who simply sought a better, cheaper high. Drug dealers found many new customers and expanded their heroin distribution efforts throughout the United States. Operating in small cells, dealers delivered heroin directly to customers on demand, making it very easy for people to consume and become addicted to the drug. Consequently, heroin use reached its highest peak in twenty years in 2016 and was responsible for the most drug-related deaths in 2015.

Yet another surge in opioid-related deaths began in 2013 with the rise in popularity of fentanyl (and its analogues) within the illicit drug market. Fentanyl, a synthetic opioid pain reliever used to treat severe pain, is thirty to fifty times more potent than heroin. Because the illicit version is easy to reproduce and inexpensive to manufacture, small amounts can equate to big profits for drug dealers—motivating many to increase their distribution of the drug. However, many users are unaware of the strength of fentanyl or unknowingly consume lethal doses of it when it is mixed with heroin or other drugs. In 2016 fentanyl surpassed heroin in the number of opioid overdose deaths, making it the deadliest drug in the United States.

A Public Health Emergency

Following the rapid increase in opioid-related deaths over the past twenty years, the US government declared opioid abuse a public health emergency in October 2017. Changing public health policy is crucial to preventing deaths and helping those who are struggling with opioid addiction. According to the World Health Organization, only 10 percent of people worldwide who need treatment for opioid dependence are receiving it. Failing to treat opioid addiction increases the likelihood that overdose rates will remain high.

Government and health officials have put forth several initiatives intended to address the opioid epidemic, including improving access to treatment and recovery services, promoting the use of drugs that reverse overdoses, creating better public health surveillance to better understand the epidemic, supporting cutting-edge research on pain and addiction, advancing better practices for pain management, and including mental health professionals in treatment plans to address psychological conditions that co-exist in people suffering from addiction. These efforts require not only widespread support from the public and the medical community but also federal funding to put needed programs in place.

To this end, in September 2018 the US Department of Health and Human Services (HHS) awarded over $1 billion in grants to fight America's opioid crisis. "Addressing the opioid crisis with all the resources possible and the best science we have is a top priority," says the department's secretary, Alex Azar. "The more than $1 billion in additional funding . . . will build on progress we have seen in tackling this epidemic through empowering communities and families on the frontlines."[2] It remains to be seen whether these efforts will work, but Americans are beginning to realize the scope of the opioid problem and take action to protect their loved ones from falling into addiction.

Chapter One

The Scope of Opioid Addiction

Like other drug addictions, opioid addiction is a chronic disorder of the brain, and anyone can suffer from it. It affects people of all ages, from all ethnicities, and from any socioeconomic status. However, the opioid crisis has struck certain areas and groups of people more than others. Regardless of the individual or the place where the person lives, the consequences of addiction are severe: Opioid use can ruin people's lives and result in their death. In fact, opioids killed nearly forty-eight thousand Americans in 2017.

What Does It Mean to Be Addicted to Opioids?

Opioid addiction or opioid use disorder (the clinical term for opioid addiction) refers to the problematic use of opioids that causes a person significant physical, mental, and emotional distress. It is a chronic illness of the brain that is characterized by intense, uncontrollable, or compulsive cravings for the drug. People are said to be addicted when they are unable to stop or control their use of opioids, despite serious and harmful consequences that result from their use, which include (but are not limited to) social problems with family and friends and an inability to fulfill work, school, or home obligations. When people become addicted, they feel as if they cannot live without the drug, and their entire world revolves around satisfying their desire for it. Efforts to stop taking opioids often result in withdrawal—characterized by physical and psychological symptoms that result from removing opioids from the body—and relapse (returning to drug use after an attempt to stop).

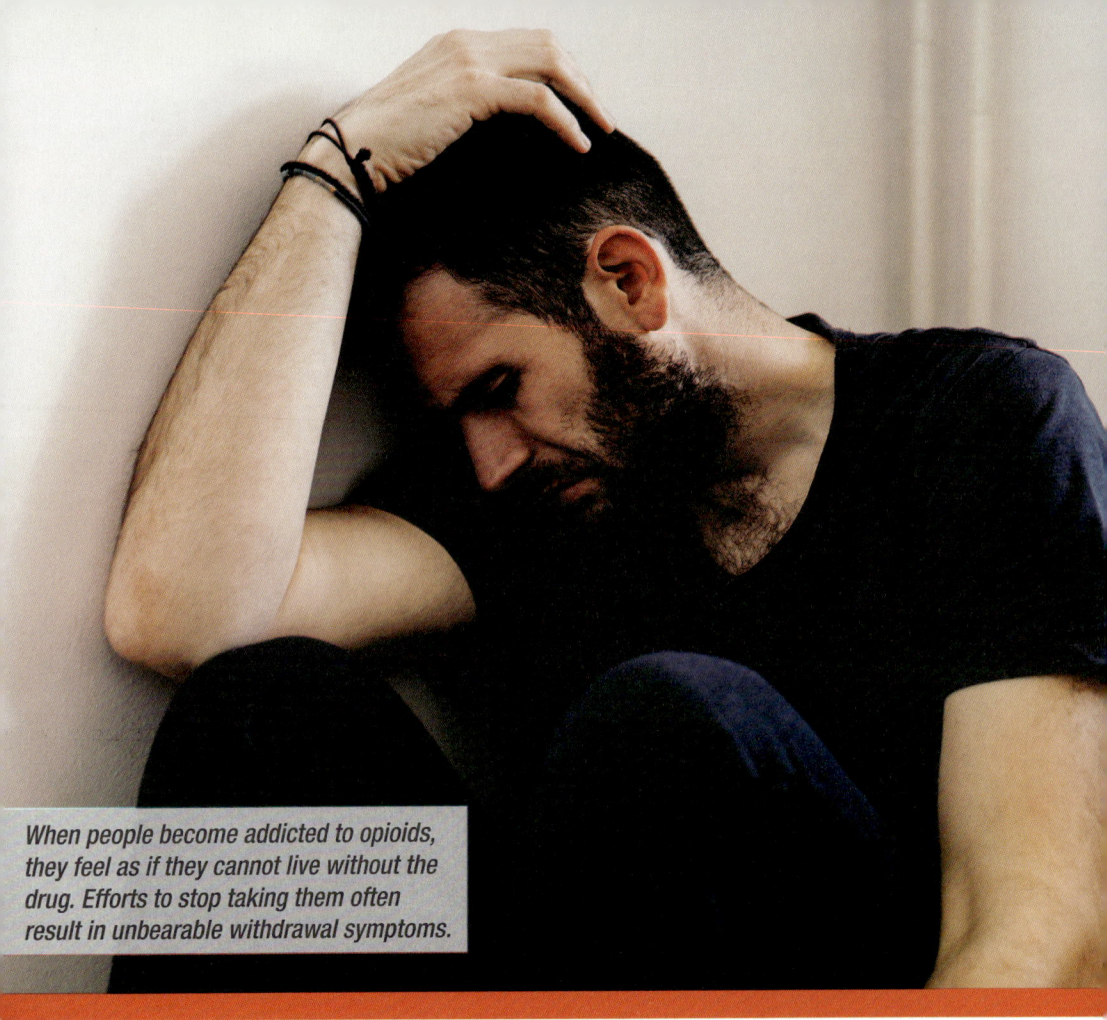

When people become addicted to opioids, they feel as if they cannot live without the drug. Efforts to stop taking them often result in unbearable withdrawal symptoms.

Many people become addicted to opioids, especially prescription opioids, accidentally. What starts out as simply taking meds prescribed by a doctor after a surgery or injury leads to tolerance (taking higher doses to feel the effects of the drugs), which often leads to dependence (experiencing withdrawal symptoms when not taking opioids) and then addiction. Others may experiment with prescription painkillers, heroin, and fentanyl recreationally at first but then become addicted after repeated use.

There are many signs that a person is addicted to opioids. Some people may find themselves taking their pills far longer than necessary to treat pain, while others may begin to need more opioids than initially prescribed to achieve the desired effect. Or some may find that they cannot successfully cut back on use. If a person spends a lot of time using, trying to get, or recovering from use of opioids, he or she is likely addicted.

Signs of Opioid Abuse

Opioid addiction typically sets in after a period of misusing opioids. At first it may be difficult to know with certainty if someone is misusing opioids. However, some common indicators include changes in normal routines, physical health and appearance, relationships, and behavior. For instance, a person might miss a lot of work or school, lose interest in activities he or she once loved, or perform poorly on the job. With regard to physical health and appearance, a person might gain or lose weight, have red eyes, lack energy and motivation, or suddenly lose interest in clothing, grooming, or overall appearance.

Sometimes drastic behavior changes occur. Relationships with family may become difficult, and friendships may end. People may become secretive and not explain where they have been or with whom they have been spending time. Individuals may lash out in anger when questioned about changes in behavior. A teenager might not allow family members into his or her room. Repeated requests for money or missing money or items from home might also point to potential drug use. A parent of a heroin addict from Payson, Arizona, describes how her son turned to stealing to fuel his heroin addiction: "It makes you do things you never would have done before. My son stole family heirloom jewelry given to me by my parents, brought here from Italy, irreplaceable. It broke my heart to tell my mother what my middle son did."[3]

> "It makes you do things you never would have done before."[3]
>
> —Parent of a heroin addict from Arizona

How Widespread Is Opioid Addiction?

People all over the world use opioids. However, according to a 2017 United Nations report, the United States ranks highest when it comes to opioid consumption. Indeed, use in the United

States is 50 percent higher than in Germany and two thousand times greater than use in India. In 2017 doctors wrote more than 191 million opioid prescriptions for patients in the United States. As for heroin, approximately 948,000 Americans reported using the drug in the past year, according to a 2016 National Survey on Drug Use and Health study.

While overdose deaths are relatively easy to track, it is difficult to know exactly how many Americans suffer with opioid addiction because many have not officially been diagnosed in a health care setting or may not be receiving care from a physician. However, in 2016, more than 11.5 million people self-reported misusing opioids in the previous year, and 1.9 million reported being addicted to the drug. Current estimates from HHS put the number of addicted people at over 2.1 million. That number is likely to be much higher, given that opioid addiction is underreported and undertreated.

Certain regions of the United States have been more heavily impacted by the opioid crisis than others. These include Appalachia, parts of the West and Midwest, and New England. According to the National Institutes of Health, the states with the highest number of opioid deaths in 2016 were West Virginia, New Hampshire, Ohio, and Maryland, as well as Washington, DC. In West Virginia, for example, approximately forty-three of every one hundred thousand people died from an opioid-related drug overdose. West Virginia was also among the top three states dispensing the highest number of opioid prescriptions in 2015, with 110 prescriptions written for every 100 people.

Interestingly, different regions have preferences for different kinds of opioids, likely due to the availability of a given drug. For example, China White, a type of heroin, and fentanyl are more common on the East Coast; meanwhile, oxycodone is more prevalent in the Midwest, and black tar heroin, a sticky dark-colored form of heroin that is less refined than powder heroin, is more widely used on the West Coast. Heroin sold in the Northeast, Midwest, and mid-Atlantic states is more often mixed with fentanyl than in other parts of the country.

A Pain Reliever with a Long History

For thousands of years, opium, a psychoactive substance derived from the seedpod of the opium poppy, has been used for medicinal and recreational purposes. Opium first became available in the United States in 1775. During the Civil War in the 1860s, doctors used morphine, the most active substance in opium, to treat soldiers for pain. It is estimated that forty thousand soldiers became addicted to the drug as a result.

Morphine and heroin, which is a morphine derivative, were commonly used for pain management in the late 1880s and early 1900s. In subsequent decades people also began to use opioids recreationally, prompting the government to limit their use to prescriptions under the Harrison Narcotics Tax Act of 1914. Due to the stigma associated with these highly addictive drugs, doctors mostly avoided prescribing them for chronic pain until the 1970s, when a renewed focus on pain management led many doctors to prescribe them for painful chronic diseases like cancer. Soon many brands of opioid painkillers arrived on the market. The three popular opioids often prescribed today—Vicodin, OxyContin, and Percocet—were approved by the US Food and Drug Administration (FDA) in the 1980s and 1990s.

Among these regions, rural areas have experienced some of the highest rates of opioid prescriptions, opioid-related hospitalizations, and drug overdose deaths. The number of opioid overdoses in rural counties saw a fivefold increase from 2000 to 2016. The crisis tends to hit areas with fewer employment opportunities, higher poverty, and limited access to health care and substance abuse treatment. Further, physicians tend to have fewer resources for pain management and usually prescribe opioids more heavily.

Despite the prevalence of opioid abuse in rural communities, urban areas are not immune from the crisis. Of large cities, Philadelphia has the highest rate of overdose in the country. An estimated seventy-five thousand residents are addicted to opioids in Philadelphia, with the neighborhood of Kensington operating as a hub for heroin distribution. In 2017, 236 people died by overdose in that neighborhood alone. Despite concentrations in certain areas, the

> "No area of the United States is exempt from this epidemic."[4]
>
> —Anne Schuchat, principal deputy director of the CDC

opioid epidemic extends across the United States. Principal deputy director of the CDC Anne Schuchat says, "No area of the United States is exempt from this epidemic—we all know a friend, family member, or loved one devastated by opioids."[4]

Who Is Most Vulnerable to Opioid Addiction?

Anyone can become addicted to opioids: they can be young, old, female, male, rich, or poor. Well-known public figures such as actor Philip Seymour Hoffman and musicians Prince, Tom Petty, and Mac Miller have recently succumbed to opioid overdoses. Addiction has no boundaries, as explained by an anonymous person treating people for addiction in South Carolina:

> Addiction does not discriminate. It is not only the "junkie" you see on the corner, begging for change who is affected. I've helped treat everyone from an Ivy League graduate from a prominent, well respected family, to an elderly Southern matriarch who became addicted after being prescribed opioids for years.[5]

While people from all walks of life are susceptible to opioid addiction, it has impacted white, non-Hispanic Americans the most. In one study, whites were 50 percent more likely than blacks and 167 percent more likely than Hispanics to die of a drug-related overdose, in part because the white population receives the bulk of opioid prescriptions. However, even though whites currently have the highest mortality rates, the CDC found an increase in opioid-related deaths for all races, with the greatest relative increase impacting the black population. The rate of fatal drug overdoses

> "Addiction does not discriminate. It is not only the 'junkie' you see on the corner, begging for change who is affected."[5]
>
> —Anonymous treatment provider from South Carolina

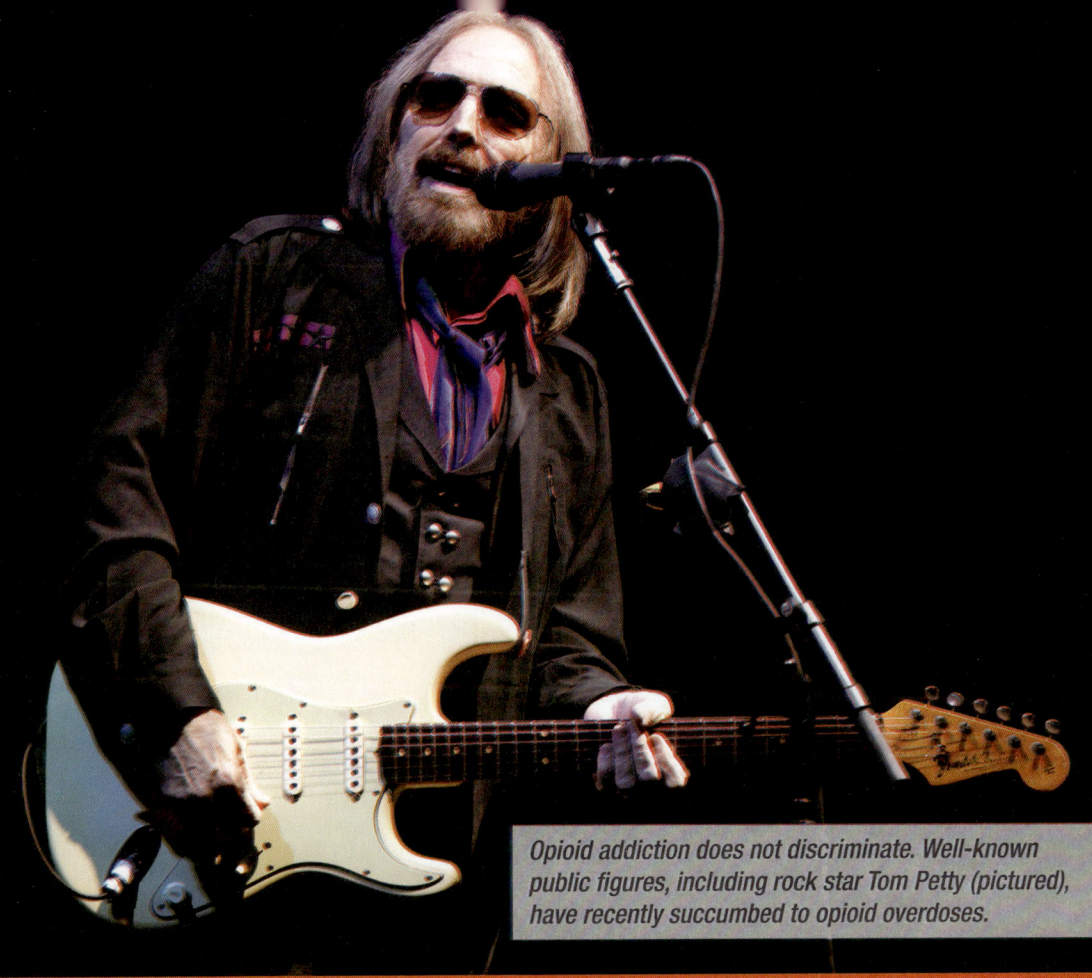

Opioid addiction does not discriminate. Well-known public figures, including rock star Tom Petty (pictured), have recently succumbed to opioid overdoses.

among African Americans has increased two times faster than fatal overdoses for whites since 2014. One of the reasons for this uptick is the presence of fentanyl and its analogues in urban areas, which have a higher density of black people. In 2017, for example, 70 percent of the 279 fatal overdoses in Washington, DC, were due to fentanyl, and African Americans accounted for 80 percent of the victims. As the nature of the epidemic changes, so do the groups of people most affected.

When it comes to gender, three times more men than women die from opioid overdose, since more men use potent drugs like heroin and fentanyl. Men are also more likely to use drugs by themselves, which increases their risk for overdose. Women, on the other hand, report more chronic pain and anxiety than men

Opioid Overdose Deaths Keep Rising

Overdose deaths caused by opioids reached an all-time high in the United States in 2017. The sharpest increase in opioid-related deaths in 2017 resulted from the synthetic opioid fentanyl. Overdose deaths from heroin and prescription painkillers have also increased, although not as steeply.

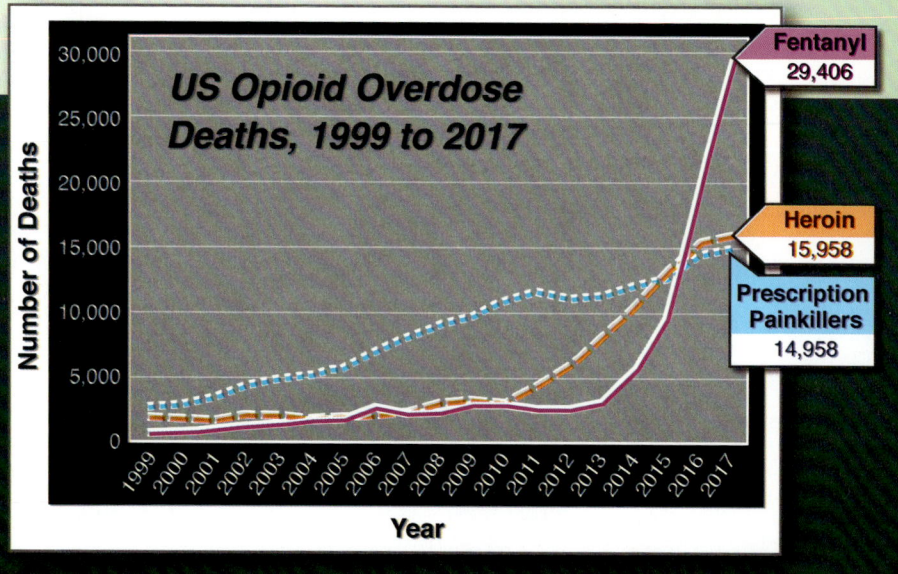

Source: National Institute on Drug Abuse, "Overdose Death Rates," August 2018. www.drugabuse.gov.

and may be more likely to self-medicate with prescription opioids. While women and men develop addictions at the same rate, women tend to give in to cravings and relapse more often than men.

Individuals in their twenties and thirties have been the hardest hit by the opioid epidemic, though all age groups suffer to some degree. Peak rates of addiction occur for women around age twenty-four and for men around age twenty-five, with addiction rates picking up again for both genders in their mid-thirties. By 2016 opioids were responsible for one in five deaths for people aged twenty-four to thirty-five, with many of those deaths due to fentanyl or its analogues.

Adolescents are particularly vulnerable to developing an opioid addiction. In a report from the CDC, 25 percent of adolescents who misused prescription opioids by age thirteen developed an addiction at some point in their life. Teens are vulnerable because their prefrontal cortexes—the part of the brain that helps people assess situations, keep emotions and desires under control, and make sound decisions—are developing throughout adolescence. Opioids impinge on teens' normal brain development, compromising their decision-making abilities and putting them at risk for continued use.

Consequences of Being Addicted to Opioids

Regardless of a person's socioeconomic status, race, gender, or age, opioid addiction has far-reaching consequences. It alters a person's brain chemistry, affects his or her psychological health, creates innumerable social and financial problems, and strains relationships with friends and family. However, death due to overdose is the most significant consequence.

Every day more than 130 Americans die of an opioid overdose. According to data from the National Institute on Drug Abuse, more than twenty-nine thousand fatal drug overdoses in 2017 were attributable to fentanyl and its analogues; this marked an increase of more than 45 percent from the previous year. The dramatic increase of drug overdose in general has actually decreased the life expectancy rate in the United States since 2015, as far as recent figures show—something that has not happened since World War II in the 1940s.

All opioids are dangerous in excessive amounts because they flood a person's systems and suppress the ability to breathe. Loss of oxygen can quickly lead to death. People who use drugs like heroin and fentanyl are especially at risk due to these drugs' potency—particularly fentanyl, which can suppress breathing in under a minute. It is extremely difficult to control the amount of fentanyl found in a product; it only takes the equivalent of two grains of salt to produce a euphoric buzz. Small errors in measurement—either in the illegal labs where the drug is made or among drug dealers' mixes—could mean the difference between life and death.

When Overdose Is Not a Deterrent

Elizabeth Brico, a writer in the Pacific Northwest, is in recovery from heroin addiction. Like many opioid users, she overdosed multiple times during her drug-using years. In a perverse demonstration of how people with an addiction think, she says, "The risk of overdose became part of the allure of getting high." She describes how she felt after her ninth overdose:

> I thought I was dead. My husband did too. He kept sneaking glances at me, or touching my hand, my arm, my leg —checking that I was not a ghost. I didn't feel like a ghost, though. I felt like a re-animated corpse.
>
> My hands and lips were visibly and palpably swollen. My mind felt like it was encased in fog. I remember walking outside and feeling unworthy of the sunlight. Like something grossly aberrant, something that did not belong among the living. I had never felt that way after an overdose before. . . .
>
> I know what it is to want to die—to have so little regard for life that I don't care or consider the consequences of anything I do. The other overdoses didn't scare me because I wasn't afraid of dying. Coming back from the dead though—and really feeling it—that was indescribable. I felt like I had violated a vital law. Like I had transgressed some ineffable border that I should not have been able to cross back over. I don't know why I am alive to tell this story, but I haven't touched heroin since.

Elizabeth Brico, "This Is What It's like to Overdose on Heroin Nine Times," *Tonic* (blog), *Vice*, August 15, 2017. https://tonic.vice.com.

Despite fentanyl's dangers, drug users are consuming more of it than ever. For some, the allure of fentanyl is its cheap cost and intense high. However, the high fades rapidly, leading users to inject or snort the drug more frequently, which puts them at even greater risk. Fentanyl also produces strong withdrawals, which encourages people to keep using the drug to avoid experiencing that pain. Others unknowingly consume fentanyl when it is added to heroin or black market oxycodone and other prescription pills.

This is what happened to pop musician Prince in 2016, when he died from a fentanyl overdose after consuming counterfeit pills that resembled the prescription painkiller Vicodin.

For every person who dies from an opioid overdose, as many as thirty individuals experience a nonfatal overdose. One CDC report estimates that from July 2016 to September 2017, 142,557 people—approximately 317 people per day—were treated for opioid overdose in hospital emergency departments. And that number only includes people who actually went to the hospital. In one 2016 study of nonfatal overdose among opioid users, nearly 36 percent of participants had experienced an overdose. Overdoses sometimes happen in waves, especially if a potent mix of drugs hit the illegal market. For instance, in a six-day period during the summer of 2016, emergency responders treated 174 opioid overdoses in Cincinnati, Ohio.

Opioid addiction is so powerful that many people overdose multiple times. In other words, surviving an overdose does not deter an addict from continuing to use opioids. North Carolina resident Mike Page overdosed at least three times when he was addicted to heroin. His life was saved only because he was revived with naloxone, a drug that reverses an overdose. "It's unfortunate that it took as many times as it did for me to change my life but that is the reality of this condition," he says. "For some people, one shot [of naloxone] is all they need. For others it takes multiple opportunities."[6]

Chapter Two

What Influences Opioid Addiction?

In the past, people who suffered from addiction were considered to be "morally weak" with no willpower. Addiction was seen simply as a behavioral choice.

However, advances in science and research have shown that addiction is a complex disease of the brain, one that has no single cause. Several factors contribute to whether a person becomes addicted to opioids, including environmental and social elements in a person's home, work, school, and community; behavioral choices such as how a drug is consumed; psychological issues such depression, trauma, and post-traumatic stress disorder (PTSD); and biological factors such as one's genes. The more risk factors a person is exposed to, the more likely that consuming opioids will lead to addiction.

Environmental and Social Factors

Environmental and social factors related to a person's family, friends, school, and community play a role in whether he or she develops an addiction. Studies show strong ties between a person's family situation and drug use, especially during adolescence. Not always, but in some cases, people who become addicted to opioids and other drugs come from families in which one parent is absent or there is no clear structure of authority. Without supervision, clear boundaries, rules, or role models, a young person may be more apt to experiment with drugs or turn to drugs for comfort.

People who struggle with addiction may also often come from dysfunctional families that feature strained or unhealthy relationships. Authority figures may behave violently or threaten violence as a means of control; they may put unrealistic expectations on children or may not offer emotional support. These situations often foster feelings of fear and distrust as well as a lack of safety and security. Studies show that the incidence of drug use is higher in families in which hostility is present, as compared to families in which warmth and love is shown. Further, those who develop addictions tend to have weak family connections on the whole.

Living with parents or other family members who use drugs or alcohol increases the risk that a child will have drug problems in the future. Witnessing drug use in the home promotes the idea that drug use is acceptable. A child longing for attention from a parent, for example, might copy the parent's behavior either to get noticed or to bond with that parent. Further, research shows a connection between alcohol consumption within a family unit and drug addiction. In one family study, alcohol was consumed in approximately 46 percent of families in which drug addiction exists. A family's history of addiction can increase the speed at which someone becomes addicted.

A person's friends also influence his or her likelihood of using and becoming addicted to drugs like opioids. When teens lack a strong bond with their parents, siblings, or caregivers, they may be more likely to make choices based on what their peers think and do. Peer pressure refers to a feeling that a person must do the same things or adopt the same beliefs and values as one's peers in order to be accepted, liked, or respected by the group. Teens often feel the greatest social pressure to conform, and many may do things they would not have otherwise done on their own. To fit in, adolescents may try a drug if the people around them are also doing drugs. Research shows that while young people think about the risks and rewards when making decisions, they are more likely than adults to favor the reward and ignore the risk—especially in situations in which friends or peers are present. According to national data, almost 50 percent of teens ages twelve to seventeen who misuse opioid painkillers got them from a friend or relative. In general, the more exposure people have to drugs within their community—whether at school or in other places that they spend time—the more opportunity they have to try and use drugs.

Behavioral Factors

The type of drug individuals choose to use, how they take that drug, and how often they consume it—that is, their behaviors surrounding or regarding a drug—influence their likelihood of becoming dependent and addicted. Because many factors influence addiction, it is not possible to say exactly how addictive a particular drug may be. However, researchers do look at several indicators to determine a drug's addictive qualities, which include how high a person gets from the drug, how quickly tolerance builds and how much more of a drug is required to get the same effect, how likely a person is to seek out more of the drug, how hard a drug is to quit, how severe the withdrawal symptoms are, and how likely a person is to relapse once addicted. Considering these factors, researchers regard opioids as highly addictive.

How people engage with a drug can also increase their risk for addiction. For example, injecting drugs like heroin and fentanyl causes them to enter the bloodstream and brain in seconds, which produces an intense high. But the intensity of the high does not usually last for more than a few minutes, which drives some people to take more in order to achieve that euphoria again. Basically, the more drug a person consumes, the more likely he or she is to become addicted to it. Someone who takes a prescription opioid pill occasionally, for example, has less of a chance of becoming addicted than someone who takes multiple pills every day.

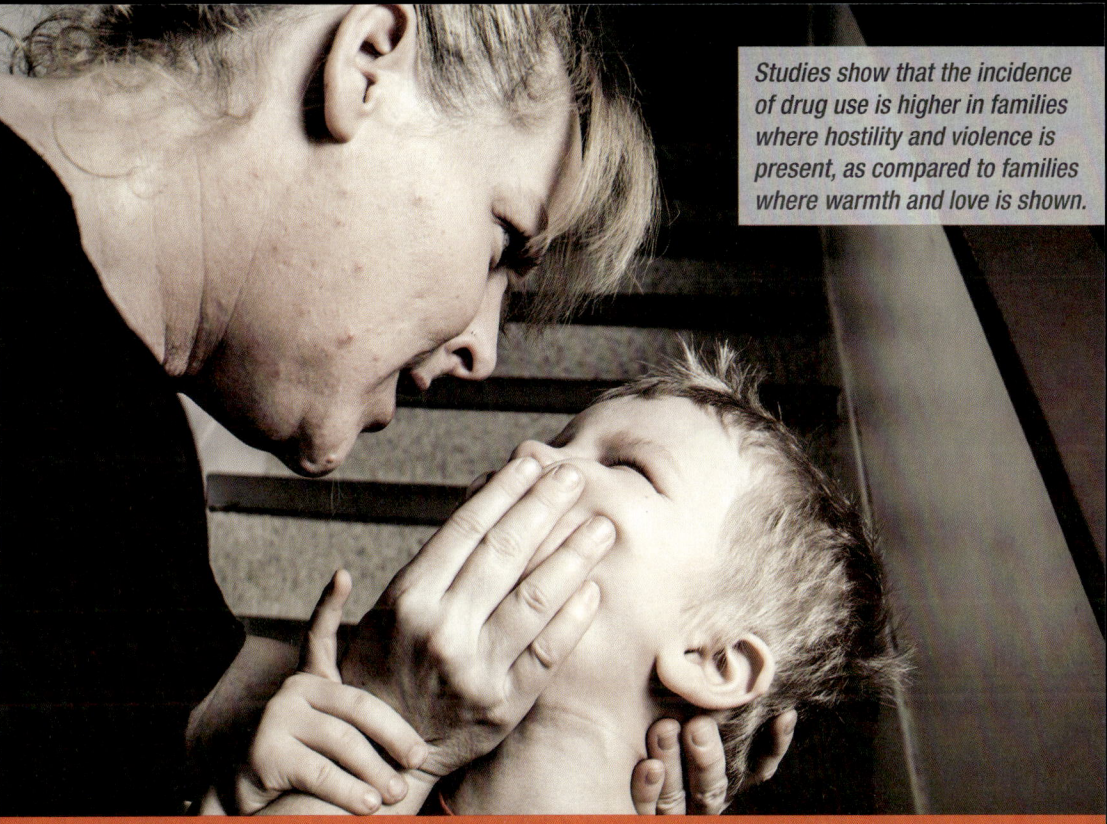

Studies show that the incidence of drug use is higher in families where hostility and violence is present, as compared to families where warmth and love is shown.

Psychological Conditions

Those who struggle with opioid addiction also tend to experience other mental issues, such as anxiety, attention-deficit/hyperactivity disorder, bipolar disorder, and depression. Doctors use the term *comorbidity* to describe a person who has two or more disorders or illnesses. The term also suggests that the interactions between the two disorders can make them both worse. For instance, many people who have an opioid addiction also have another mental illness, and many people who are diagnosed with a mental illness of some sort often end up misusing drugs. It is estimated that about 50 percent of people who are diagnosed with one will develop the other during their lives. Many teens and young adults who have an opioid disorder tend to also have anxiety or depression.

A strong correlation exists between opioid use and depression. Scientists believe that depression doubles the likelihood a person will use opioids, while opioid use doubles the likelihood that a person will develop depression. Researchers at Saint Louis University found that 10 percent of one hundred thousand patients (or ten thousand people) who had been prescribed an opioid for ailments such as back pain, arthritis, and headaches developed depression after one month of taking the medication. These patients had not been diagnosed with depression prior to treatment. Conversely, many people suffering with depression turn to opioids to alleviate their symptoms—such as persistent feelings of sadness or loss of interest in life—but prolonged use of opioids seems to enhance those very same feelings.

For many people with mental illness, opioids offer a refuge from physical and psychological trauma, economic disadvantage, social isolation, and hopelessness. People with mental ill-

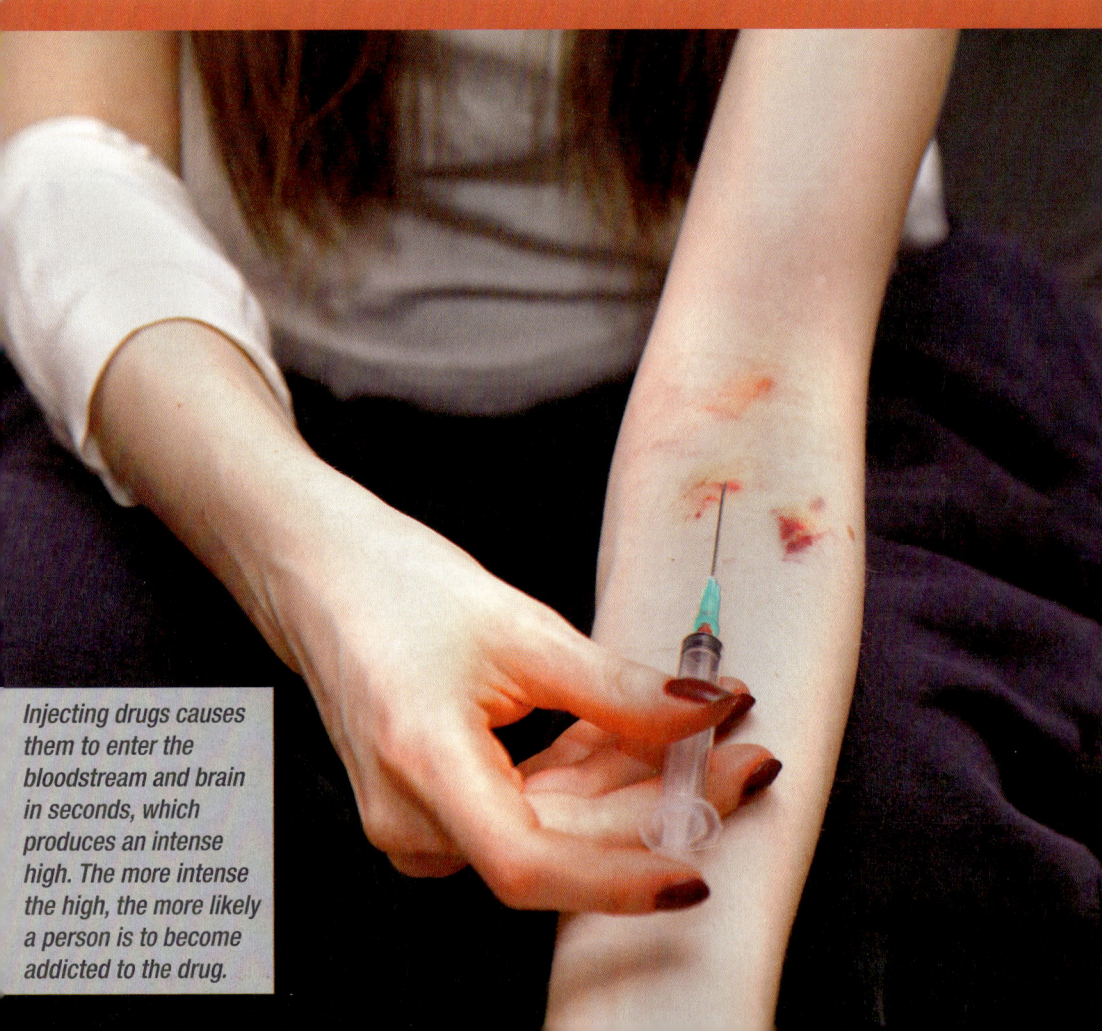

Injecting drugs causes them to enter the bloodstream and brain in seconds, which produces an intense high. The more intense the high, the more likely a person is to become addicted to the drug.

ness may self-medicate with drugs in order to cope with painful feelings like anxiety, alienation, and loneliness. Researchers estimate that 48 percent of heroin addicts experience some form of depression, usually triggered by feelings of hopelessness, despair, and guilt that arise from their drug use. However, the more individuals rely on opioids to relieve their other symptoms, the more dependent they become on them for relief, which encourages continued use and creates a cycle of use and abuse. Karen Boland describes how her son's untreated depression turned into an opioid addiction: "Cory died of his addiction, but he also died because the medical profession failed him. Please don't think that I feel my son had no responsibility for his death. He absolutely did, but so did all the doctors who overprescribed medications without getting to the root of his problem: depression."[7]

> "Cory died of his addiction, but he also died because the medical profession . . . overprescribed medications without getting to the root of his problem: depression."[7]
>
> —Karen Boland, mother who lost her son to a heroin overdose

Trauma and PTSD

People who experience a traumatic physical or psychological event sometimes develop a condition called PTSD. The experience varies from person to person, but some of the most common traumatic events involve childhood physical and sexual abuse, sexual assault, violent assault, natural disasters, and military combat. Individuals who suffer from PTSD often experience tremendous stress or anxiety, intrusive memories, intense flashbacks, insomnia, aggressive behavior, and angry outbursts. People with PTSD may experience the symptoms at any time, especially when they are reminded of the traumatic event.

PTSD develops when individuals have not fully processed or resolved their feelings associated with the traumatic event. This emotionally debilitating condition can interfere with daily life, since

The Myth of the Addictive Personality

Does someone's personality determine whether he or she will develop an addiction? The idea that a single personality type leads to addiction is a myth that is often perpetuated by images portrayed in the media. For example, the "fiendish criminal" or the "antisocial loner" do not accurately describe a lot of people who become addicted to drugs. In fact, a vast array of personality traits can contribute to addiction; how these play out are dependent on a wide range of environmental, behavioral, psychological, and genetic factors.

Journalist Maia Szalavitz writes about the myth of the addictive personality in her book *Unbroken Brain*:

> Research finds no universal character traits that are common to *all* addicted people. Only half have more than one addiction (not including cigarettes)—and many can control their engagement with some addictive substances or activities, but not others. Some are shy; some are bold. Some are fundamentally kind and caring; some are cruel. Some tend toward honesty; others not so much. The whole range of human character can be found among people with addictions, despite the cruel stereotypes that are typically presented. Only 18% of addicts, for example, have a personality disorder characterized by lying, stealing, lack of conscience, and manipulative antisocial behavior. This is more than four times the rate seen in typical people, but it still means that 82% of us don't fit that particular caricature of addiction.

Maia Szalavitz, *Unbroken Brain: A Revolutionary New Way of Understanding Addiction*. New York: Picador, 2016, pp. 58–59.

individuals often feel powerless and out of control. In order to gain a sense of control and/or numb the pain they feel, those with PTSD may use drugs as a way to escape. Elizabeth Brico self-medicated with heroin to cope with the symptoms of PTSD she developed after being abused by an older man for four years.

> It was years since I had last been in contact with my abuser, but living with post-traumatic stress disorder is like being stuck in time. On heroin, time moved forward. Off heroin,

I was seventeen and being beaten endlessly. It seemed to me then, as the agony of recovery grew nearer, that I was better off strung out.[8]

According to the National Center for PTSD, the most common cause of PTSD and addiction for women is sexual abuse, while military combat often causes PTSD and addiction for men. For instance, from 60 percent to 80 percent of Vietnam War veterans needing treatment for PTSD also require substance abuse treatment. Bessel van der Kolk, medical director of the Trauma Center at the Justice Resource Institute and a professor of psychiatry at Boston University, explains how trauma can easily lead to an opioid addiction. "Trauma is about your fight/flight response going crazy. Morphine blocks that fight/flight response, so your body gets quiet and you don't get stuck in fight or flight."[9] Consequently, opioids

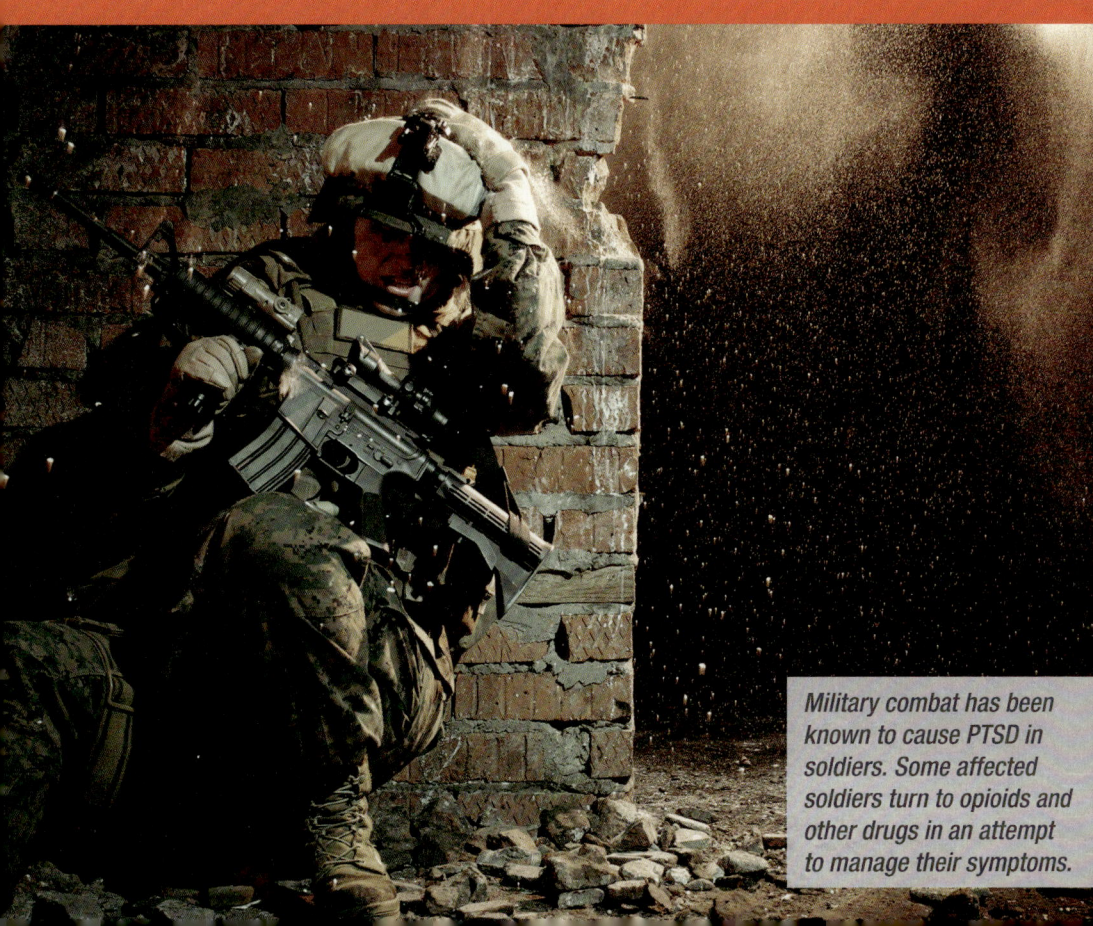

Military combat has been known to cause PTSD in soldiers. Some affected soldiers turn to opioids and other drugs in an attempt to manage their symptoms.

provide significant relief for people suffering with PTSD, which is why many get hooked on them.

Role of Genetics

Scientists believe that genes also play an important role in addictive behavior. Genes are the basic hereditary units by which a parent transfers information about certain traits and characteristics to an offspring. Certain genes can make people more or less likely to develop an addiction in the same way that genes influence a person's risk for other diseases like cancer or diabetes. Therefore, the risk of a person developing an addiction increases when a blood relative, such as a parent or sibling, also has an addiction to drugs. The National Institute on Drug Abuse estimates that a person's genes, including the impact of environmental factors on how those genes function, may account for 40 percent to 60 percent of a person's risk for addiction. For instance, a parent's stress and trauma can cause genetic changes that can be passed on to children. These altered genes may then increase the chances the child will later develop a substance abuse disorder.

So far, scientists have found it challenging to identify the exact genes responsible for opioid dependence because genes are not the sole reason a person becomes dependent or addicted. However, researchers from three prominent universities recently identified a gene that could be tied to opioid addiction. In a study of more than three thousand patients exposed to opioids, researchers found an alteration, or variant, near the RGMA gene, which is located in cells in the frontal cortex of the brain and tells nerve fibers where they need to go. Those patients with the variant were more likely to have symptoms associated with opioid dependence. It is possible that the

> "We believe this is a good new lead and hope it encourages novel pharmacological approaches to treating opioid dependence."[10]
>
> —Joel Gelernter, a doctor and researcher at Yale University

Addiction and Attachment Anxiety

Attachment theory refers to an inborn system that takes root during infancy. The quality of care a child receives during early life, such as a caregiver's sensitivity and response to the child's signals, can determine how that child relates to others throughout his or her life. Attachment anxiety is a fear of being abandoned, and it typically develops when attachment figures (such as parents or other caregivers) are not present, are inconsistent, or are unpredictable during the formative years. Babies are born with the desire to be close to a caregiver and to feel safe in dangerous or uncertain situations. If babies experience neglect, abuse, or confusing responses, they may find it difficult to regulate their emotions. As a result, they may develop insecurities that manifest in various ways in their relationships.

Anxiously attached people may struggle with substance abuse. They may take drugs in order to cope with the stress of an underlying insecurity. Or they may turn to drugs to avoid painful emotions and to detach from psychological distress. Choosing drugs creates a "chemical shortcut" to avoiding intense emotions such as pain and frustration. However, this behavior can easily become habitual. Self-medicating only provides temporary relief from these negative feelings, which can magnify feelings of loneliness and emptiness. Thus, people repeat the substance abuse in order to not feel those emotions.

---

genetic variant disrupts the brain's nerve circuits and changes the way the brain responds to opioids. Whether a person feels good taking a particular opioid might be influenced by the way the genes are expressed.

While there is much to be learned about the role of genetics in opioid addiction, scientists' discoveries offer clues that could help make prevention and treatment efforts more effective. For instance, scientists could develop a drug that targets the RGMA gene and protects people from the onset of an opioid addiction. According to Joel Gelernter, a doctor and researcher at Yale University and senior author of the RGMA study, "We believe this is a good new lead and hope it encourages novel pharmacological approaches to treating opioid dependence."[10]

Chapter Three

How People Become Addicted to Opioids

When people first take opioids, most do not plan on taking them for months or years. Some begin taking them via legal prescriptions for pain, assuming they will only be on them for a few days or weeks. Others may experiment with opioids recreationally, curious about the effects or wanting to fit in with others. During these initial stages of use, people are not immediately reliant on the drugs to function physically and mentally.

With repeated use, however, they develop a tolerance to opioids and eventually become dependent on them to function normally. Eventually, opioids are incorporated into their normal routines, and drug use begins to disrupt their life. At this point, addiction sets in, and they feel as if they cannot live without the drug. They will do almost anything to continue its use regardless of the consequences. "Having an opioid addiction is like having a full-time job that you never have a break from,"[11] says one fentanyl user from Calgary, Canada.

Misusing Opioid Prescriptions

Every day, over 25 million Americans experience chronic pain. More people experience pain than cancer, heart disease, and diabetes combined. People feel pain for a variety of reasons, including after complicated surgeries, during and after childbirth, following serious injuries, and for other medical conditions. Many more experience regular migraines, backaches, and neck aches. In fact, pain is one of the most common reasons people visit their doctor every year.

Chronic pain refers to pain that lasts at least three months or beyond the time it normally takes the body to repair tissues. For many people, pain persists for years. Doctors often regard chronic pain as a disease in itself because it impairs a patient's well-being, quality of life, and ability to function. Treating pain is difficult, which is why doctors often prescribe opioids. According to the CDC, more than 17 percent of Americans were given at least one opioid prescription in 2017, with an average of 3.4 prescriptions per patient. How long opioids are prescribed varies from person to person and depends on the person's level of pain. However, while opioids may alleviate pain for a time, they do not cure its source.

> "Having an opioid addiction is like having a full-time job that you never have a break from."[11]
>
> —A fentanyl user from Calgary, Canada

One of the ways an opioid addiction begins is by misusing legal opioid prescriptions. Because opioids can so effectively mask pain, it can be difficult to stop taking them once a person starts. Additionally, because opioids also make people feel calm, happy, and relaxed, a person can quickly become accustomed to this new state of being. As a result, some patients ignore the recommended dosage and take more than they should or continue to use the drug even after their physical pain subsides. According to the CDC, 11.5 million Americans misused prescription opioids in 2016. In some cases those who no longer take their prescriptions sell or give their excess pills to others. According to one study, approximately 33 million Americans—10 percent of the total population—have reported using opioids recreationally during their lifetime. The reason behind the high number of recreational users is that many people believe that opioid painkillers are safer and less addictive than heroin and other illicit drugs.

The first time Randi, a former opioid addict from Portland, Oregon, used prescription painkillers was after she injured her back at work. At the emergency room, doctors prescribed her medication for her pain. "I soon found that I liked them," Randi says. "I

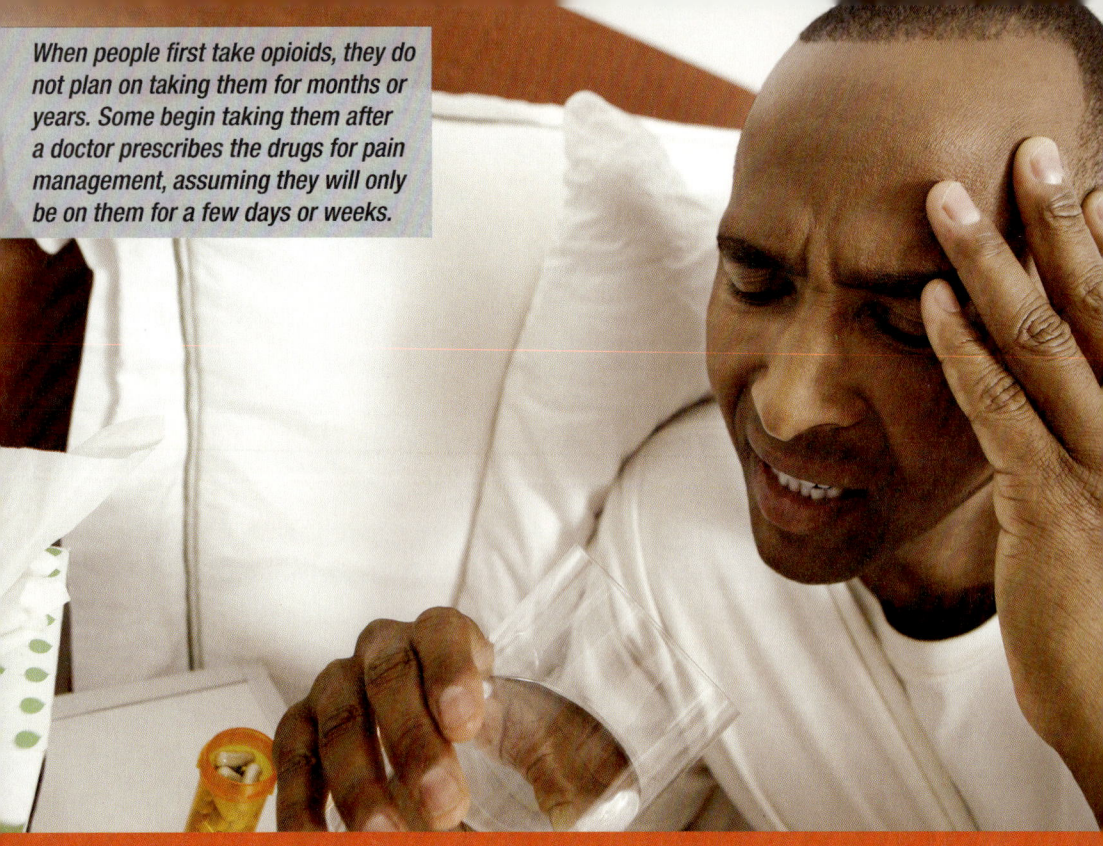

When people first take opioids, they do not plan on taking them for months or years. Some begin taking them after a doctor prescribes the drugs for pain management, assuming they will only be on them for a few days or weeks.

knew they were easy to get at that time. So all I had to do was say I was in pain and then I would get unlimited prescriptions. And that went on for a couple of years. . . . At one time I was getting a prescription for 90 percoset a week."[12] Like many others who have misused prescription opioids, the ease with which Randi could get pills eventually led her to become addicted.

Triggering the Brain's Reward Center

Regardless of the type of opioid—prescription painkillers, heroin, or fentanyl—all opioids mimic the pain-relieving effects of chemicals that are produced naturally by the body. As opioids are absorbed into the bloodstream, they seek out opioid receptors in the nerve cells located in the brain, spinal cord, and peripheral nervous tissues. These receptors help balance mood and regulate stress responses. Once the opioids attach to the receptors, they block the body's pain signals. At the same time, the opioids stimulate the brain's reward center, causing it to release dopamine, a chemical messenger known as a neurotransmitter. Dopamine invokes feelings of pleasure and euphoria—or the high associated with opioids—which are transmitted to the body via the nervous system.

Dopamine signals to the brain that an important event has happened; it is also produced when a person experiences intense pleasure through acts such as eating, drinking liquids, having sex, and taking care of babies, all of which are necessary for human survival. Dopamine tells the brain a desirable activity has taken place and needs to be repeated. Every time opioids are consumed, dopamine is produced, which reinforces the value of taking them. The problem with opioids, however, is that they cause the body to release dopamine in excessive amounts. This excess dopamine is far greater than what the body needs to derive pleasure or sustain life.

Changes in Brain Chemistry

These chemical reactions alter a person's brain over time. As the body monitors its chemical levels, it adjusts its own production of natural opioids to manage what is being added. In other words, if the body receives a lot of opioids externally, it decreases production of natural opioids to protect against overstimulation. Additionally, people who use large amounts of opioids for a long time reduce their body's response to the chemical. So a person taking opioids may need higher quantities of the drug to feel the same effects. When this happens, a person has reached a state of tolerance. Tolerance allows an opioid user to handle a dose ten times larger than a dose that would kill a nonuser of opioids.

Dopamine surges also disrupt the body's natural system and start to rewire circuits in the brain. The body stops regulating dopamine in the way it once did. Feelings of stress, anger, or dissatisfaction set in without the opioids, which encourages a person to take more to cope with the uncomfortable feelings. As a result, the dopamine system becomes more responsive when opioids are present.

Addiction Is Not Chosen

Most people do not choose to become addicted to opioids. Lynn, who has been sober for six years, describes how little choice plays a part in addiction. She says addiction is a process that takes place over time:

> I wish people understood how much I wanted to stop, how much I hated what my life had become. I think people assume that there is a lot more choice involved than there is. But I don't think anyone really chooses to become a heroin addict. I chose to start getting high initially but . . . by the time heroin came into the picture it was too late, I was already gone. Heroin does not sound like a good idea to a rational human being and some people can use other recreational or prescribed drugs and remain rational. Those of us who become junkies are people who are rendered incapable of making good decisions when mind-altering substances are introduced to our bloodstream. You might call it a slippery slope, the regression from casual partying to heroin but it's really a very slow process of accepting different levels of normality.

Quoted in *Frontline*, "Heroin & Opioid Addiction, In Your Own Words: Lynn Who Has Been Clean for Six Years." http://apps.frontline.org.

Eventually, a person derives less and less pleasure from the drug but craves it all the more. The brain adapts to these levels and demands more of the substance to try to re-create those extremely pleasurable feelings that came from initially using the drug—sometimes referred to as "chasing the dragon." This is particularly true for heroin users, who may take hundreds or thousands of doses hoping to feel the euphoria they felt the first time they took the drug.

These chemical changes in the brain cause a person to behave differently, bringing out characteristics like impulsivity and impaired decision-making as well as repetitive and self-destructive behavior. At this stage the brain's reward pathways are wired for drug-seeking and drug-taking behavior. Ultimately, the brain begins to operate normally when opioids are present but abnormally when the drug is no longer present in the system.

Opioid Dependence and Withdrawal

As people transition from voluntary to habitual use of opioids, they are said to be dependent. Opioid dependence is often coupled with tolerance and happens when the body adapts to the presence of opioids in its system. If a person either reduces the amount of the drug or stops taking it, the body experiences unpleasant physical and psychological symptoms known as withdrawal.

During long-term opioid use, the body adjusts to the high level of opioids in its system and designs ways to flush the toxic substances from the body. However, once the opioids are removed from the system, the body does not immediately adjust, resulting in physical side effects, or withdrawal. These physical symptoms include stomach cramps, nausea, aches and pains, sweating with chills, muscle spasms, rapid heartbeat, insomnia, and seizures. They can start a few hours after last taking opioids and

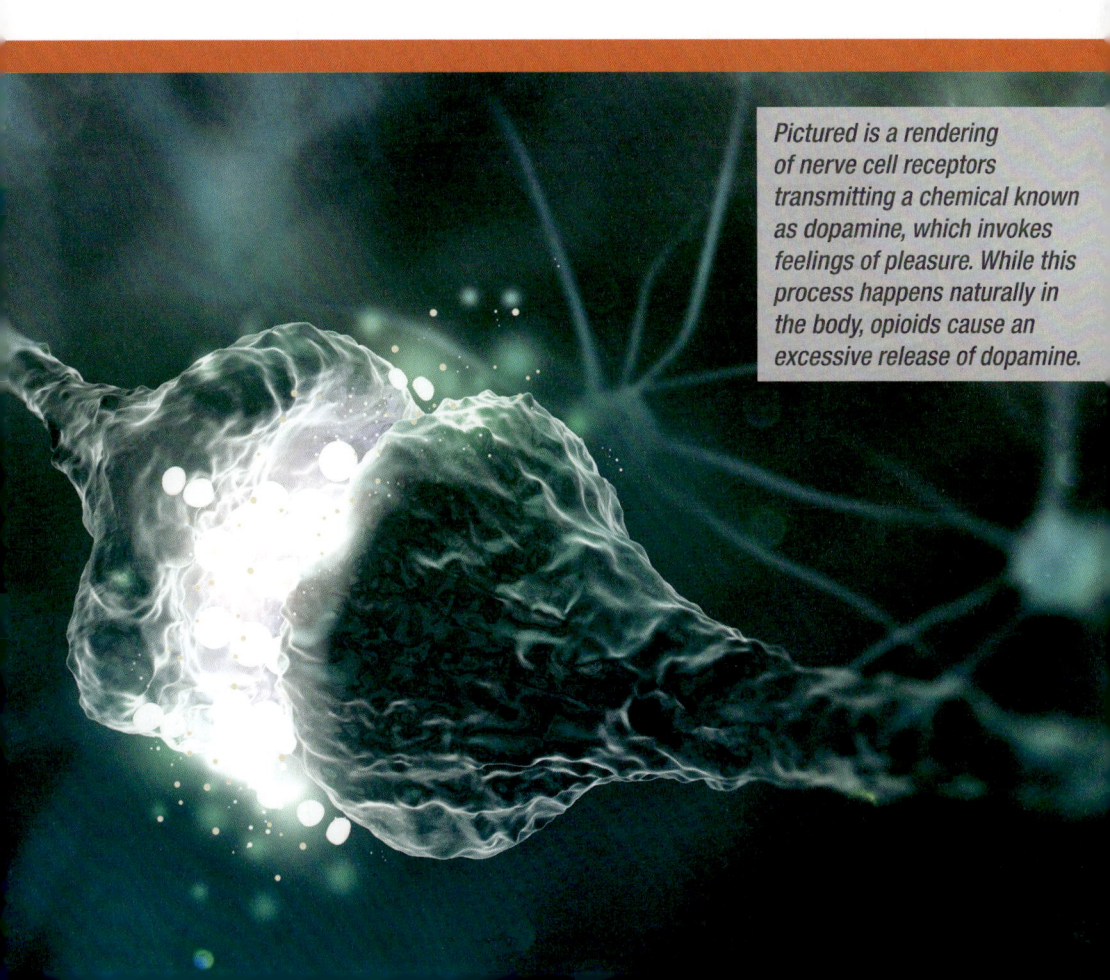

Pictured is a rendering of nerve cell receptors transmitting a chemical known as dopamine, which invokes feelings of pleasure. While this process happens naturally in the body, opioids cause an excessive release of dopamine.

occur for up to ten days. Doctors often compare many of these symptoms to a bad flu. The severity of these symptoms can vary greatly among people, even among those with similar gender, body size, and dosage levels. Rocco Merolli took OxyContin for four years after breaking his back and went through withdrawal when he stopped taking the medicine. "It was one of the worst experiences I've ever had," he says. "I felt like I had the worst flu I've ever had, on top of anxiety so bad I thought I could have a heart attack. Let's just say my stomach and bowels got very loose, both ways."[13]

While the physical symptoms last for days, the psychological symptoms of withdrawal can persist for weeks. A person may experience anxiety, depression, nightmares, feelings of hopelessness, and an intense desire to use opioids again. Maia Szalavitz, a leading journalist and writer on addiction and a former heroin addict, thinks the psychological withdrawal from opioids is worse than the physical withdrawal. "What makes drug withdrawal hard to take is the anxiety, the insomnia, and the sense of losing the only thing you have that makes life bearable and worth living, not the puking and the shaking," she says. "It's the mental and emotional symptoms—the learned connection between drugs and relief and between lack of drugs and pain—that matter."[14]

> "I felt like I had the worst flu I've ever had, on top of anxiety so bad I thought I could have a heart attack."[13]
>
> —Rocco Merolli, formerly addicted to OxyContin

The desire to avoid withdrawal is what drives many people to continue to use opioids and is part of the cycle of addiction. When Michelle was twenty-three and a senior in college, she broke her neck after she was pushed off a balcony and landed on her head. She spent six months in a neck brace and another six months in physical therapy while also taking a prescription opioid for the pain. She remained on the pain pills for ten years due to the fear of becoming ill once she stopped taking them.

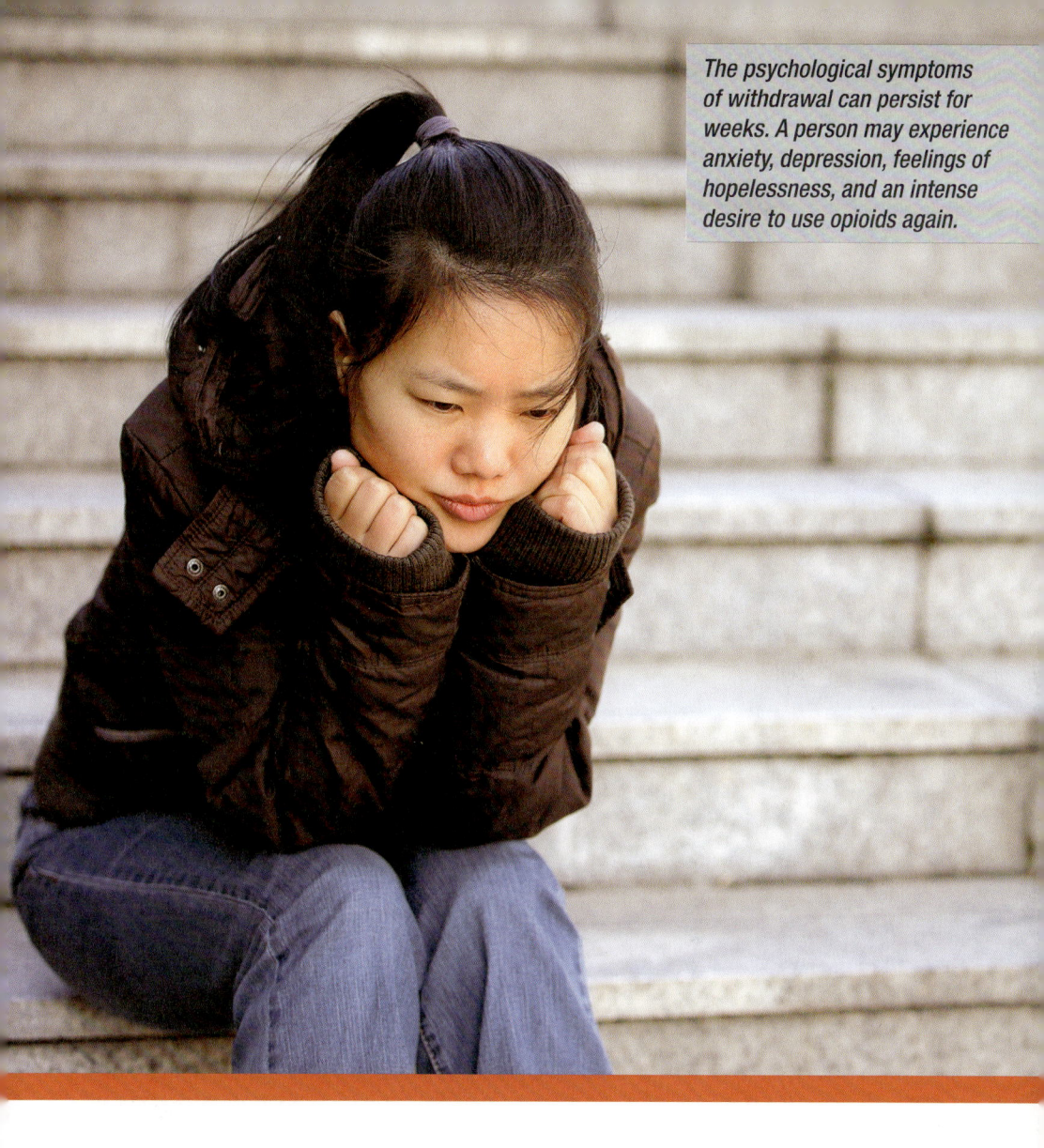

The psychological symptoms of withdrawal can persist for weeks. A person may experience anxiety, depression, feelings of hopelessness, and an intense desire to use opioids again.

Addiction and Relapse

During full-blown addiction, a person becomes consumed with getting and taking opioids in order to feel normal and be able to function. Most people suffer just to make it through the day. Many addicts are aware of their increased risk of dying by overdose. However, even that knowledge does not usually deter them from continuing to consume greater amounts of the drug. According to Sidarth Wakhlu, an addiction psychiatrist in Dallas, Texas, "It doesn't mean they're suicidal or uninformed.

Tracking Addictive Behaviors in the Brain

Scientists use neuroimaging to capture images of the body's brain and nervous system at work—and what they are learning has important implications for understanding addictive behaviors in humans. Neuroscience researchers at the National Institute on Drug Abuse have developed a miniature microscope that enables them to look inside a rodent's brain. The microscope will allow them to study how complex behaviors like addiction are tied to specific neuron activity in the brain.

Mounted on the skulls of mice and rats, the tiny microscope is roughly the weight and diameter of a penny. The rodents used in the experiment have been genetically modified to express a certain protein. The protein helps make the neurons visible to the microscope, which then records the activity of hundreds of thousands of neurons simultaneously. The microscope has allowed researchers to observe the rodent's dorsal striatum, an area that plays a role in reward and addiction. By studying these areas, researchers hope to gain a better understanding of the complex interactions between brain neurons and circuits during addiction behaviors. These findings could lead to the development of new prevention and treatment approaches down the road.

It's the nature of addiction. Addiction is powerful, cunning and baffling."[15]

Given how powerful an opioid addiction can be, it is very difficult to recover from one, even if a person would like to. Like other chronic diseases, addiction is subject to periods of relapse—when someone who had stopped using opioids for a period of time decides to begin using them again. Relapsing is not inevitable, but many people with opioid addiction relapse multiple times. According to the National Institutes of Health, relapse rates are between 40 percent and 60 percent, which is similar to relapse rates for those addicted to alcohol or cocaine.

People relapse for many reasons, but among the most common is the belief that they have gained control over their drug use and can stop if their use gets out of control. Depression and the longing for opioids make people susceptible to relapse too, especially when they are weak or in pain and the cravings become too difficult to ignore. After an awful experience of withdrawal alone in a motel room in Mexico, Dr. Marc Myer, a drug treatment provider and former opioid addict, relapsed immediately upon returning home to the United States. He says, "I felt so awful, so dehydrated, overwhelmed with feelings of cravings to use again just to feel better. I got off the airplane, immediately went to an emergency room and complained of headache and other pain symptoms so that I could get opioids."[16] Some people may encounter the people and places associated with their opioid use, which triggers strong feelings to use again. Lastly, it can be mentally exhausting to learn how to manage life day in and day out without opioids. Ivana Grahovac, a forty-two-year-old from California, describes how easy it is to slip back into using again: "That old impulse comes back, that old habituated response, which is: 'This is hard. You're going to fail. Don't even try to get well. You're just going to end up back in it. So just go get high right now.'"[17]

> "Addiction is powerful, cunning and baffling."[15]
>
> —Sidarth Wakhlu, an addiction psychiatrist in Dallas, Texas

Chapter Four

Living with Opioid Addiction

People addicted to opioids are living with a chronic disease much like cancer. Opioid addiction is a disease they face every single day, and it influences almost every aspect of their lives. It not only takes a serious physical, psychological, and economic toll on users, it also impacts their relationships with friends, family, and peers, as well as greater society.

A Physical Toll

While opioids provide pain relief along with pleasurable sensations, they also take a physical toll on the body. Individuals who are intoxicated by opioids experience several physical symptoms, such as slurred speech, constricted pupils, and extreme drowsiness. They usually have a short attention span and may experience memory problems. The immediate physical effects will disappear as the drug dissipates in the body.

Someone who takes a large single dose of an opioid may experience severe respiratory distress and overdose. When individuals overdose, their breathing slows, they experience an irregular heartbeat, the body starts to shut down, and fluid starts to back up in the airways. Other symptoms include shallow or erratic breathing; loss of consciousness; a choking sound in the throat; discolored lips and fingernails; a blue or gray complexion; vomiting; a limp body; and slow or no pulse. A person overdosing on fentanyl may have muscle spasms or a locked jaw. It is critical that someone experiencing these symptoms get medical assistance immediately; otherwise, the person could die.

When opioids are used for an extended time, they can cause serious long-term damage to the body. Opioid use impacts the brain and liver, as well as the body's nervous, digestive, endocrine, respiratory, circulatory, and immune systems. Just a few of the long-term physical effects include a loss of coordination or a slowing of physical movement; nausea, uncontrollable vomiting, abdominal distention, and constipation; liver damage; reduced levels of hormones like estrogen and testosterone; damage to the mucous membranes in the nose, throat, and upper lungs; collapsed veins; and compromised immunity.

Opioids particularly impact the circulatory system. Heroin is often cut or diluted with additives such as sugar, starch, or powdered milk, which can become trapped in small capillaries and clog the blood vessels leading to the lungs, brain, kidneys, and liver. The loss of blood flow to these major organs can cause severe damage. These substances may also carry infectious particles or bacteria that enter the bloodstream and can cause endocarditis, an inflammation of the lining of the heart. In one study, people who used OxyContin were twice as likely to have a heart attack as were non-opioid users. Injecting opioids for long periods can lead to inflammation and abscesses at injection sites. Over time veins become weak and may eventually collapse.

Despite the serious physical toll of long-term opioid use, the body can recover from many of these conditions over time if a person stops using opioids. Veins will start to heal when heroin is no longer injected, inflammation will subside, and hormone levels will begin to normalize. How much someone heals is dependent on each person's overall health, but most people will experience some physical improvement.

Increased Risk of Disease

Many opioid users who inject heroin, fentanyl, or crushed prescription pills may use shared or "dirty" needles, which can quickly

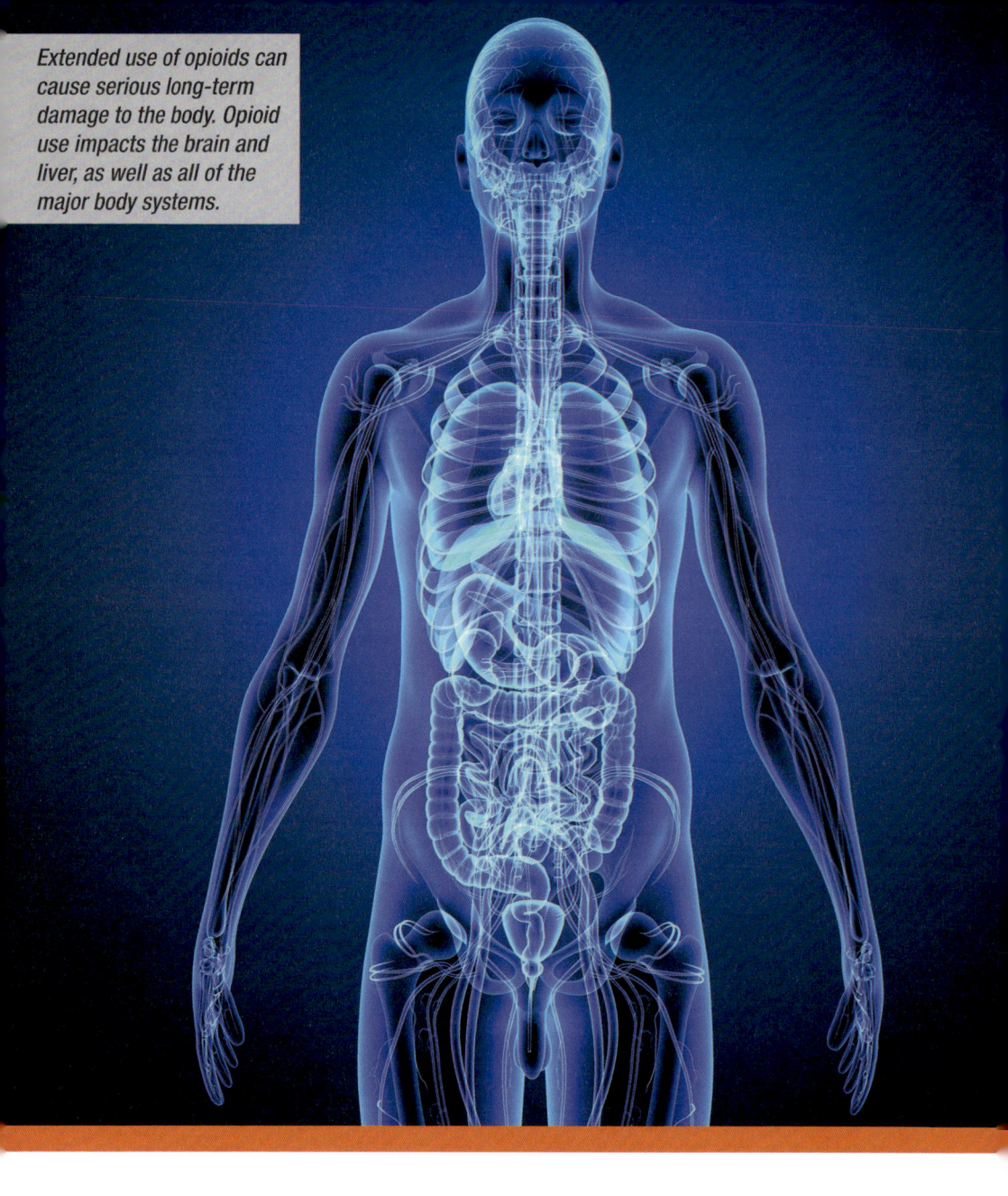

Extended use of opioids can cause serious long-term damage to the body. Opioid use impacts the brain and liver, as well as all of the major body systems.

transmit potentially deadly diseases from one person to another. Some of these diseases include HIV, tetanus, tuberculosis, and hepatitis B and C. People who inject opioids have a high risk for contracting the hepatitis C virus, a potentially deadly infectious disease that killed twenty thousand Americans in 2015. Hepatitis C infects the liver, and if left untreated it can lead to liver failure, liver cancer, and cirrhosis. According to the CDC, from 2010 to

2015, cases of hepatitis C tripled, mainly as a result of increased opioid use. Michigan liver specialist Dr. Robert Fontana comments on the uptick in hepatitis C cases: "We see at least one or two patients a month coming into our hospital with an acute hepatitis C infection, and they are frequently young people who are using and experimenting with illicit drugs."[18]

While hepatitis C is curable, approximately 70 percent to 80 percent of people infected with the virus show no symptoms and are unaware that they have the disease. As a result, many unknowingly pass the disease to others via shared needles. Other people knowingly take the risk. Thirty-four-year-old Jerry Searp of Kentucky was diagnosed with hepatitis C in 2011 after shooting heroin with a friend at a house where other drug users gathered. He recalls, "I asked to use his needle and he said, 'Hey, I've got hep B and C.' . . . And at the time it didn't really matter to me. The desire to get high was just so great."[19]

Because addiction lowers people's inhibitions, individuals might engage in unprotected sex, which further puts them at risk for disease. Others may even trade sex in exchange for opioids, and still others may pass a sexually transmitted disease along to their spouse or partner. Pregnant women who abuse opioids are at risk of transferring certain viruses like HIV to their unborn child in utero. Babies may also be born addicted to opioids and can experience withdrawal symptoms, which can be fatal for a newborn.

A Psychological and Emotional Toll

Severe changes in mental health and behavior occur in someone who is struggling with addiction. Some of the psychological changes include poor judgment, agitation, apathy, and a loss of sense of self. Individuals often struggle to recognize the dangerous situations they put themselves in, such as driving while intoxicated, engaging in abusive relationships, consuming lethal doses of drugs, or not knowing what is actually in their drugs (like fentanyl-laced heroin).

Most individuals do not choose to become addicted to opioids. Most would like to stop the addiction but feel they have no control over it. When they fail repeatedly at stopping, they start to internalize that failure, which creates a negative cycle of self-hatred. The idea that someone can stop at any time negates the fact that to be able to exert self-control, a person needs the part of their brain that regulates self-control to be functioning properly.

People addicted to opioids often have trouble relating to and connecting with other people. It becomes increasingly difficult to interact with others, which leads opioid users to isolate themselves. As the compulsion to use opioids progresses, an addict

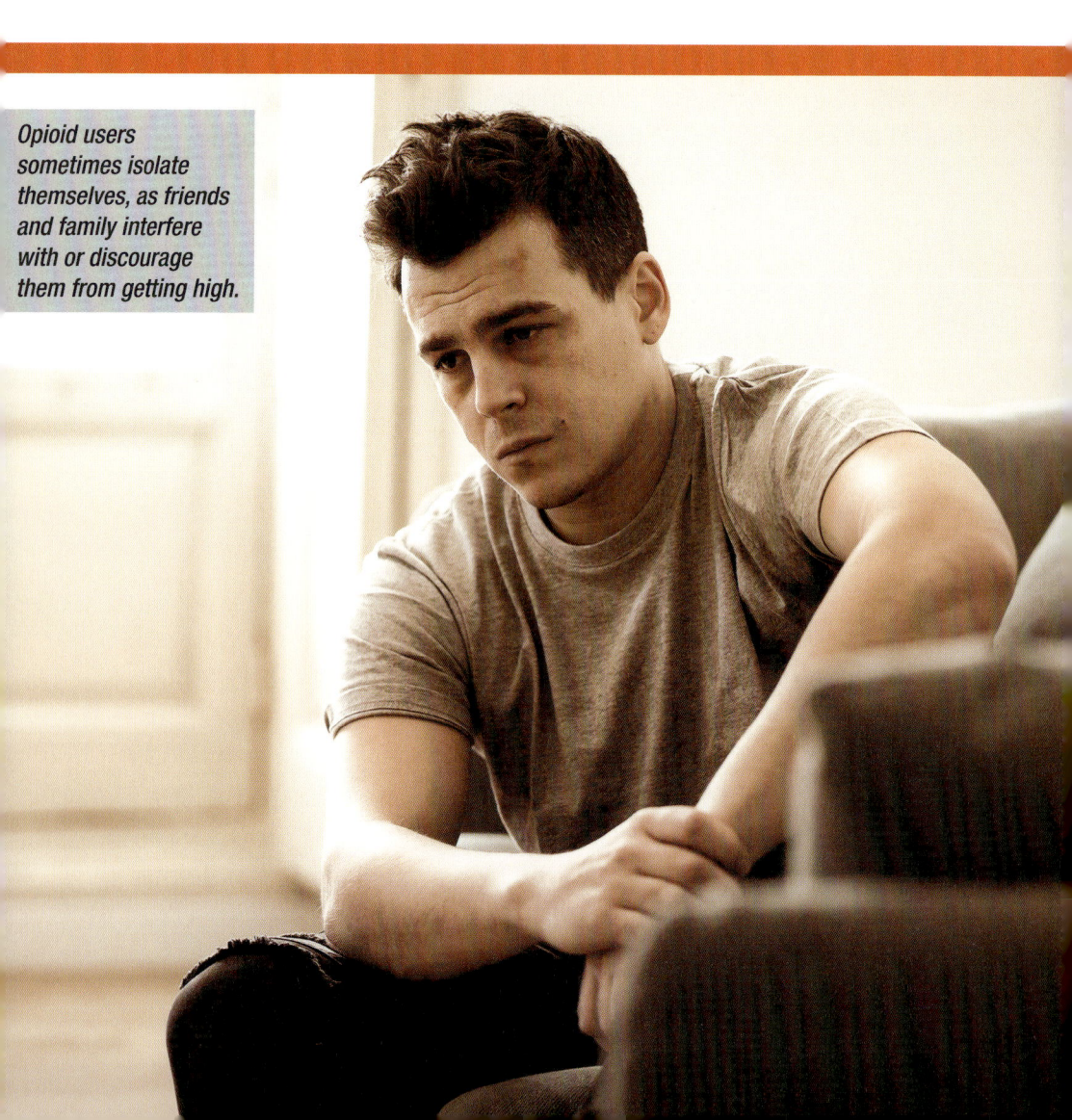

Opioid users sometimes isolate themselves, as friends and family interfere with or discourage them from getting high.

will typically detach from anyone who might get in the way of their drug use. Nobody can compete with their desire to get high or escape reality. One former user of fentanyl pills describes his self-imposed isolation: "A little pill was controlling me. Like it literally took over my mind, my thoughts, to where I pushed my wife away, my kids."[20]

> "Anything that comes in between our addiction is the enemy."[21]
>
> —Niko McManus, a mental health counselor

Further, when addicted people are alone, they can escape criticism from others who say they should not be doing what they are doing. Isolation is dangerous because an addicted person avoids potential intervention from others that could initiate treatment and recovery. Mental health counselor Niko McManus describes how isolation is a dangerous component of addiction:

> We continue to reinforce the lies that the drug is telling us. The drug tells us we need it, that we cannot survive without it. In order to keep that outlet in our lives, we have to shut everyone and everything else out of our hearts and minds. It's amazing what tricks addiction can play on us, like a master manipulator separating us from any lifeline around. Anything that comes in between our addiction is the enemy.[21]

People also find themselves isolated after damaging relationships with friends and family members. Many individuals express anger and verbal and emotional abuse toward loved ones in order to cover up their feelings of fear, denial, and guilt associated with their opioid use. These behaviors eventually push people away, and users often find themselves alone—not only physically but also emotionally and spiritually. Users may be left feeling sad, hopeless, and abandoned and without anyone to talk to or understand them. This loneliness only tends to perpetuate their drug use. Journalist Susana Ferreira describes how people's relationships with themselves and others lies behind most drug use: "An individual's unhealthy relationship with drugs often conceals frayed relationships with loved ones, with the world around them, and with themselves."[22]

Toll on Family and Friends

Opioid-addicted people's behavior impacts more than themselves; their negative behaviors can be felt by family, friends, and their community. Parents with an opioid addiction are often not available or present for their children, who may feel neglected and ignored and act out at school. Children may even mimic the habits of their parents and develop their own drug addictions. An addicted person may lie or steal, creating a climate of distrust and stress within the family. Relationships with friends often become strained as the addicted person focuses his or her energy on the addiction. Mandy McCandless, a twenty-three-year-old from Pennsylvania, describes how her addiction led her to use people: "I felt like all my relationships were very surface-level, and really I was holding people hostage. No one was really my friend. I just wanted to take things from them."[23]

> "An individual's unhealthy relationship with drugs often conceals frayed relationships with loved ones."[22]
>
> —Journalist Susana Ferreira

Family and friends may blame themselves for not being able to help the addicted person. Sometimes addiction can trigger others to become enablers and caretakers as they take over the responsibilities of the addict or cover up the addict's behavior in order to protect him or her. For example, enablers might lie to people about the person's drug use, blame others for poor behavior, or not directly address the addicted person to avoid conflict. Taking on these roles puts undue pressure on them and can lead to their own mental health problems (such as depression or anxiety) as they focus so much of their energy on the addicted person and ignore their own needs. Caregivers often face many burdens associated with a family member's drug use. In one 2013 study of

New York City Sues Opioid Manufacturers

In early 2018 New York City filed a $500 million lawsuit against eighteen opioid manufacturers and distributors to recoup some of the costs associated with the deadly opioid epidemic. Over one thousand people in New York City died of an opioid-related drug overdose in 2016—the highest year on record. The following year the city logged forty-five thousand emergency room visits related to opioids. Costs mounted for expanded opioid treatment services, hospital stays, medical examiners, criminal justice, law enforcement, and naloxone overdose programs, creating a financial burden for the city.

New York City district attorney Michael E. McMahon explains the impact of the crisis and the reason for the lawsuit:

> The reckless decision to push highly addictive prescription pills on an unsuspecting public undoubtedly led to the heroin and fentanyl epidemic that is currently devastating Staten Island, the city, and the entire country. Given the lives, hours, and resources that have been put into this fight, it is long overdue that we hold the manufacturers and distributors accountable for the people and families that have been destroyed by opioids. . . . Many of the earliest victims of this drug epidemic fell prey to the misleading and deceptive marketing behind these pills and the unchecked supply that flooded our communities for years. Tragically, nothing can be done to bring back the loved ones we have already lost, but the actions being taken [today] will only strengthen our fight against drug abuse across the city.

Quoted in NYC, "Mayor de Blasio Announces Lawsuit Against Nation's Largest Opioid Manufacturers and Distributors," January 23, 2018. www1.nyc.gov.

family members, 99 percent of participants stated that it not only disrupted family routine but also family leisure, and 98 percent said drug use hurt family interactions.

When a person dies from opioid addiction, family and friends are often left feeling hopeless and depressed, wondering what they could have done to save their loved one. Melissa and Dale Sexton lost their twenty-three-year-old daughter, Katy, to a fentanyl overdose in October 2017. Melissa describes the emotional toll on her and her husband: "And now we are left with this huge, gaping void in our life, in our family, trying to figure out: How are we supposed to move on from this?"[24] Not only do they mourn the loss of their daughter and all that she could have been, they also grapple with feelings of guilt and failure. Dale says, "I don't know what would or could have made a difference. I just know it was my responsibility, and I didn't meet it."[25]

A Financial Burden

Addiction burdens people financially in addition to physically, psychologically, and emotionally. Addiction is expensive and often leads to financial instability for the opioid user. A drug habit that stretches over several years could cost hundreds of thousands of dollars. One man spent $100,000 or more over the course of his addiction to fentanyl. Some lose their jobs—and thus their incomes—due to their inability to function normally at work. Without an income, they can no longer pay for their rent or mortgage and bills. Those who are parents or spouses may not be able to provide for their families.

Joy, a mother and former nurse, found herself homeless as the result of an addiction to prescription opioids. She lost her job and sold most of her belongings to pay for drugs. She says, "This time last year, I had a home . . . I had a car, a house full of furniture, a lot of nice stuff."[26] Many addicts do not have the means to support their addictions over the long term and may turn to stealing money and personal belongings from others to support their habit. Worse, many move to harder, cheaper drugs, which in turn carry more serious consequences.

Another financial burden is the expensive cost of treatment. The majority of people addicted to opioids cannot afford to seek treatment. The average cost of drug rehab can range from $2,000 to $25,000 or more, depending on the type of treatment and whether it is inpatient or outpatient. The US Department of

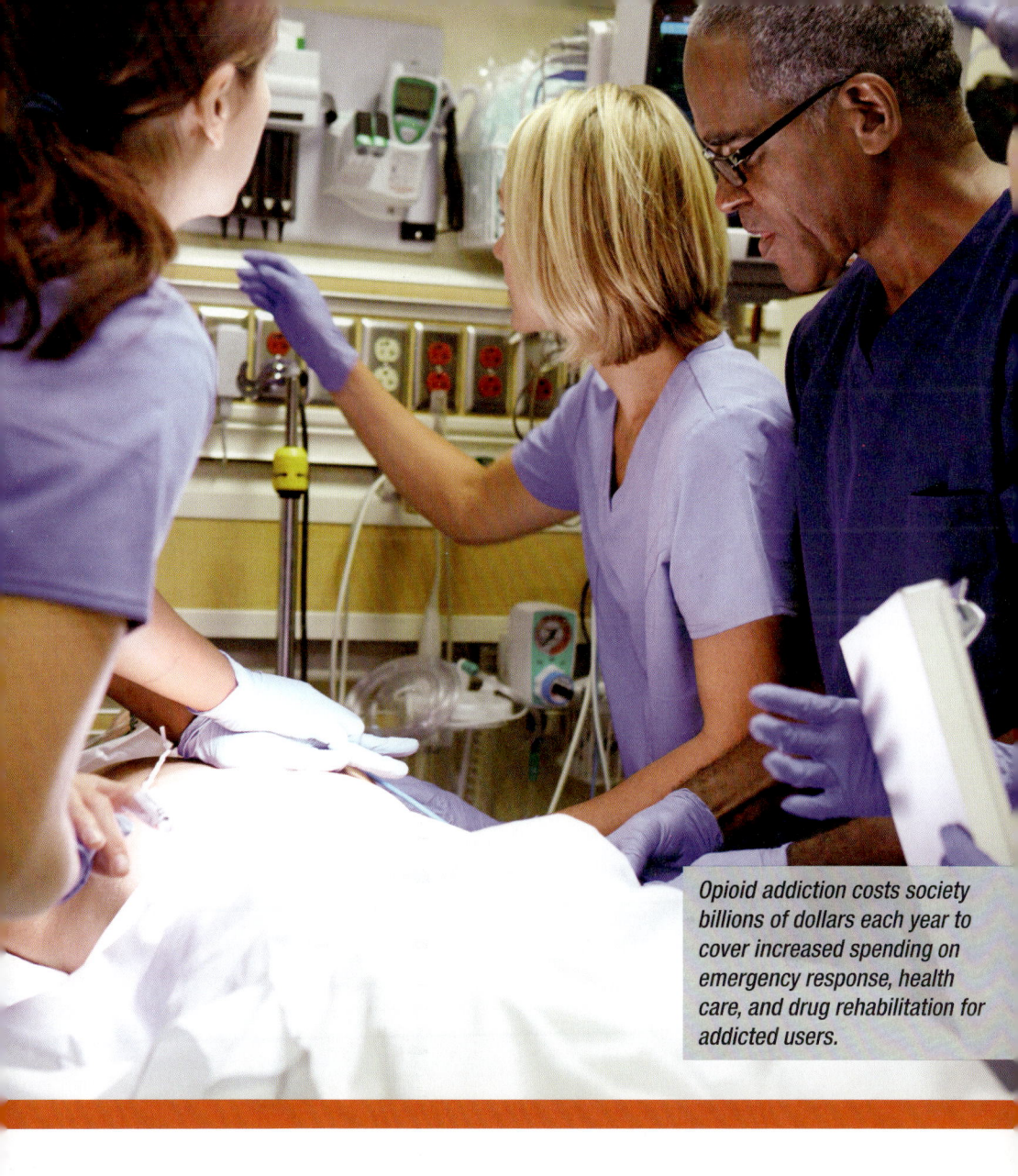

Opioid addiction costs society billions of dollars each year to cover increased spending on emergency response, health care, and drug rehabilitation for addicted users.

Defense says the cost of treatment depends on the treatment. Even for people who can afford treatment, the cost can be prohibitive, especially if a person relapses and goes to treatment multiple times. Destini Johnson's parents delayed retirement in order to pay for their daughter's several stints at rehab. After Destini's several failed attempts, the Johnsons could no longer afford treatment for their daughter, which amounted to $50,000 per month.

Opioid Epidemic Fuels Growth of the Foster Care System

Since 2010 the number of US children entering foster care has grown, coinciding with the rise of the opioid epidemic. According to a March 2018 report issued by the US Department of Health and Human Services, from 2012 to 2016 the foster care population rose by 10 percent, largely due to parents who either were addicted to opioids and unable to care for their children or had died from an overdose. In fact, substance abuse is a factor in one-third of the cases in which children are removed from their homes. In the states hit hardest by the opioid epidemic, the number of children in foster or state care has increased by 15 percent to 30 percent on average from 2014 to 2018. In West Virginia the foster care population had grown by 42 percent since 2014, largely a result of the state's high rate of opioid overdose deaths.

The increase in foster children puts further pressure on a nearly at-capacity foster care system and limited government resources. Wendi Turner, executive director of the Ohio Family Care Association, describes the situation: "Children that are coming into care are staying in care longer because there's a higher risk of relapse with their parents. . . . I don't think our state was prepared for the number of children coming into care so quickly."

Quoted in Emily Birnbaum and Maya Lora, "Opioid Crisis Sending Thousands of Children into Foster Care," *Hill* (Washington, DC), June 20, 2018. https://thehill.com.

In addition to the personal financial burdens, addiction also costs society billions of dollars each year in lost tax revenue and increased spending on emergency response, social services, health care, drug rehabilitation, and enforcement of drug laws. Much of the cost is borne by local and state governments. For example, in Dayton, Ohio, an area deeply impacted by the opioid epidemic, emergency care for opioid overdoses from 2016 to 2018 topped $1.3 million, while overdose reversal drugs like naloxone cost the city $500,000 from 2015 to 2018. It is estimated that annual costs to all levels of the government are $78.5 billion, which does not include what individuals and families have spent. Altarum, a nonprofit health care research firm, estimates that from 2001 to 2017 the total cost of the opioid epidemic was $1 trillion. The research firm projects another $500 billion in costs associated with opioid misuse, opioid use disorders, and premature mortality by 2020, especially if no sustained action is taken to address the epidemic.

Society cannot afford to ignore the opioid epidemic. Finding lasting solutions to combat the opioid crisis must take center stage to safeguard the lives of Americans battling addiction to opioids and to reduce the number of people dying from overdose.

Chapter Five

Overcoming Opioid Addiction

Addiction is a complex but treatable disease. However, it cannot be cured by simply not using opioids for a few days. Successfully treating opioid addiction requires significant time, effort, support, and resources, and thus it has proved to be an enormous challenge for many people. While some may be able to kick an opioid addiction on their own, most people require treatment to recover their lives. Effective treatment programs must help individuals not only stop using opioids but also maintain a drug-free lifestyle—one in which they can function successfully at work, within their families, and in society.

Detoxifying from Opioids

Detoxification is the first stage of addiction treatment. It is a process of allowing all of the opioids to move through a person's system without replacing them with more opioids. It is a difficult first step because a person must go through withdrawal—the very thing most opioid users want to avoid. While some individuals choose to detox at home, most physicians and treatment specialists recommend that people detox under medical supervision, especially those with a serious or life-threatening addiction. Sherry Benton, a psychology professor at the University of Florida, describes the challenge of detoxing without help: "Quitting opioids makes you so sick that you desperately want relief. Most people find it intolerable. Medical detox makes it easier to withdraw and lessens the risk of relapse."[27]

Detoxifying the body is a physically and psychologically vulnerable process. A detox facility offers a safe, clean, and supportive environment where medical professionals can intervene in the event of an emergency. Patients receive round-the-clock monitoring and care from doctors, nurses, and therapists trained in addiction-related treatments. Vital signs such as pulse rate, temperature, respiration rate, and blood pressure are checked on a regular basis. Medical staff treat and provide relief from withdrawal symptoms with over-the-counter medicines but may administer stronger medications such as buprenorphine and methadone to ease the detoxification process. Participants are encouraged to rest as much as possible. Writer and former opioid user Emily Carter Roiphe describes the importance of being in a supportive setting:

> It's very good for an addict to be in a treatment setting when they're withdrawing, because as soon as you feel physically better, the disease gets into your mind. You think: I could go for a walk and use once without all this happening again. The withdrawal doesn't do anything to remove the addiction. The addiction is still there. I don't know of anyone who all of a sudden just stopped and never went back to it.[28]

Detoxification programs typically last anywhere from a few days to two weeks. The length of the stay depends on how often a person used, any underlying medical conditions, number of substances they are detoxing from, and how long they have been misusing the substance. Following a successful detox, patients are encouraged to enroll in either outpatient or inpatient treatment programs to address the underlying causes of their addiction—because detoxification alone rarely helps patients achieve long-term abstinence.

Medication-Assisted Treatment

Abstinence-based treatment programs—meaning a person is not allowed to use opioids under any circumstances (unless for some medical procedures)—are one treatment option. However, many of these programs follow outdated faith-based models that do not take into account scientific research on addiction or the fact that opioid addiction is different from other drug addictions. Nora Volkow, director of the National Institute on Drug Abuse, believes that abstinence-only programs are not the best form of treatment for opioid addiction. "There may be some misusers for whom it does work, but in the majority of cases it does not. People with OUD [opioid use disorder] have a very high rate of relapse in abstinence-only

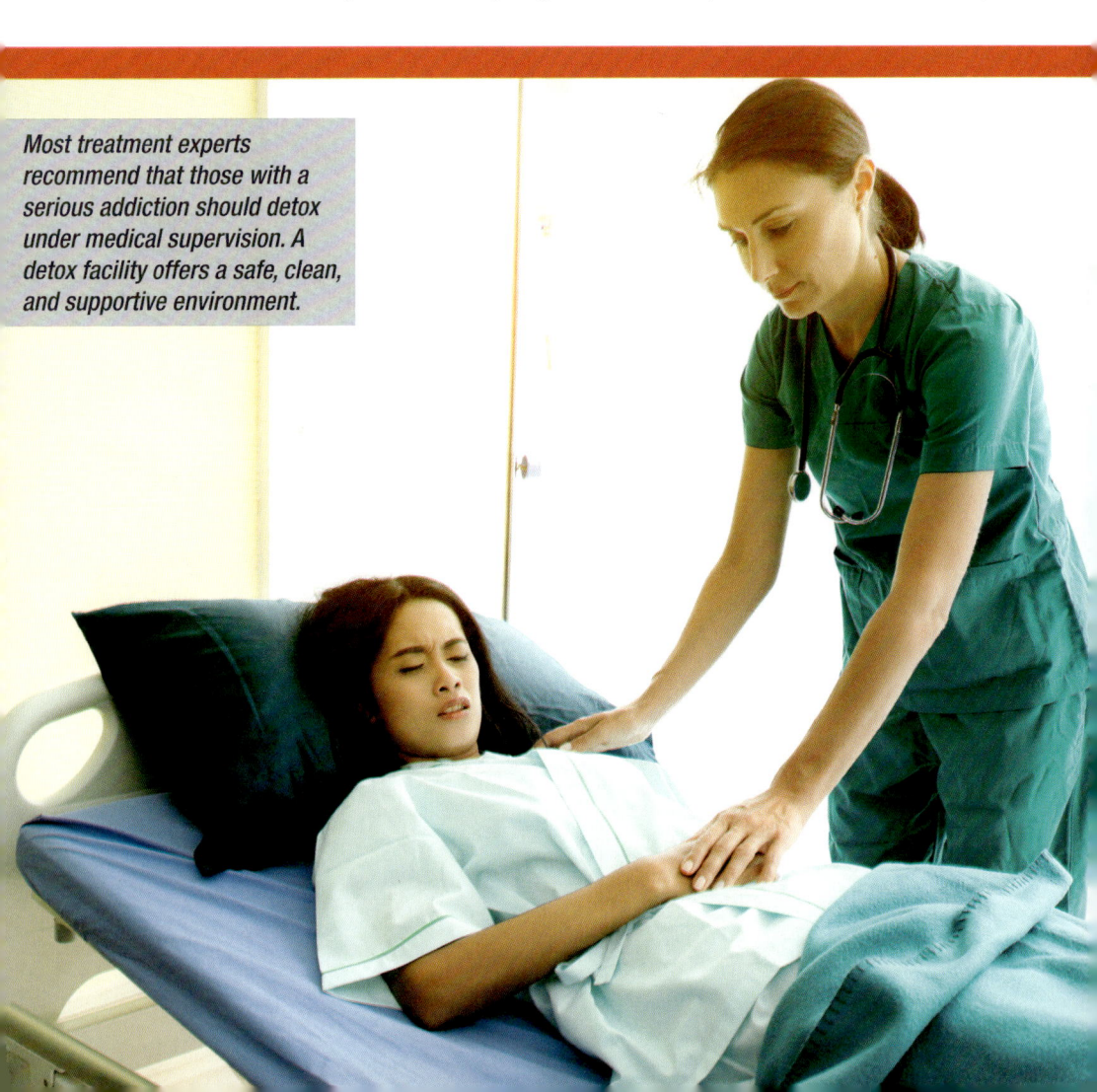

Most treatment experts recommend that those with a serious addiction should detox under medical supervision. A detox facility offers a safe, clean, and supportive environment.

programs, and the death rate during relapse can be as high as 90 percent."[29]

Given the low success rate of these programs, medications are increasingly becoming an integral part of many opioid treatment plans because they better help patients taper use and ease withdrawal symptoms. Known as medication-assisted treatment (MAT), these programs combine the use of medications with counseling and behavioral therapies that aim to treat the whole person. Two of several FDA-approved medications are methadone and Suboxone. While critics think these medications merely replace one opioid for another, the medications give people an opportunity to manage their addiction over time without going into withdrawal.

Methadone is a synthetic opioid often used as a substitute for heroin. Because it eases withdrawal symptoms, it gives drug users a break from the all-consuming daily task of getting and using heroin, allowing them an opportunity to reintegrate into society. Methadone maintenance therapy is often administered at private and public clinics regulated by state and federal laws. Treatment can last from one year to several. As part of the therapy, patients receive daily doses of methadone under a doctor's supervision. Research has shown that doses in the range of 80 to 100 milligrams per day are most effective for controlling cravings. In fact, in one study those patients receiving a higher dose of methadone were two times less likely to use heroin as were those on lower doses. Jacob, a former prescription painkiller addict and heroin user, describes how methadone helped him learn how to manage his life:

> It has helped me take everything little by little. It has allowed me to make my recovery and life changes from this long addiction manageable. My mom and dad split up recently, but I didn't use over it. . . . My life is better in every way. I have been able to focus on healing, getting my life in order and balancing out a whole new way of living and thinking.[30]

> "The death rate during relapse can be as high as 90 percent."[29]
>
> —Nora Volkow, director of the National Institute on Drug Abuse

Fentanyl Testing Strips

One harm-reduction approach that is helping prevent opioid overdose deaths consists of fentanyl testing strips. Unlike naloxone, fentanyl strips are used prior to actual drug use. The strips are dipped into the residue of cooked heroin or a crushed pill and mixture of water for at least fifteen seconds, then placed on a sterile surface. If a single line appears, fentanyl is present in the heroin or counterfeit pills. Two lines indicate a negative result.

While test strips do not identify all forms of fentanyl and do not inform users of how much fentanyl is in the drugs, they can decrease the number of overdose deaths related to fentanyl. In an October 2018 RTI International study, people who detected fentanyl in their drugs were five times more likely to change how they took their drug than were those who did not use the test strips. In fact, 56 percent of users with positive test strips decreased the amount of the drug they injected, pushed the syringe slower, snorted instead of injected, and administered a "tester" shot before consuming their regular dose. In some cases a positive result encourages users to not use the drug at all, not use alone, or use with a naloxone kit nearby.

Suboxone, a combination of buprenorphine and naloxone, is another prescription medication used to treat opioid addiction. Buprenorphine behaves like opioids but does not create the same high and is thus less likely to be abused. The naloxone portion of the medication blocks opioids from the brain's receptors, preventing the user from experiencing a high if other opioids are consumed. As a result, users tend to feel fewer psychological cravings. In fact, studies on Suboxone treatment have shown steady doses of the medication improve physical functioning. For Amanda, a former heroin user, Suboxone has helped her reclaim some normalcy in her life: "I felt like I could finally get out of bed, function and take a shower! I was impressed that my head wasn't foggy and I didn't feel 'high.' That feeling hasn't changed over time."[31]

Overall, MAT has been shown to improve survival rates, increase treatment retention, decrease the use of illicit opioids, and increase patients' ability to secure employment. Despite its success, the rate of treatment is fairly low—only 10 percent of people with opioid use disorder receive MAT. According to Richard Schottenfeld, a professor of psychiatry at Yale School of Medicine, it has been challenging for many opioid users to get help for their addiction. "Treatment hasn't been readily available. It's difficult to get, expensive and not necessarily covered by insurance,"[32] he says. While these medications might give people a better chance at recovery, they do not cure addiction alone. Along with taking medications, patients in MAT participate in behavioral therapy and counseling, usually offered through inpatient and outpatient treatment programs.

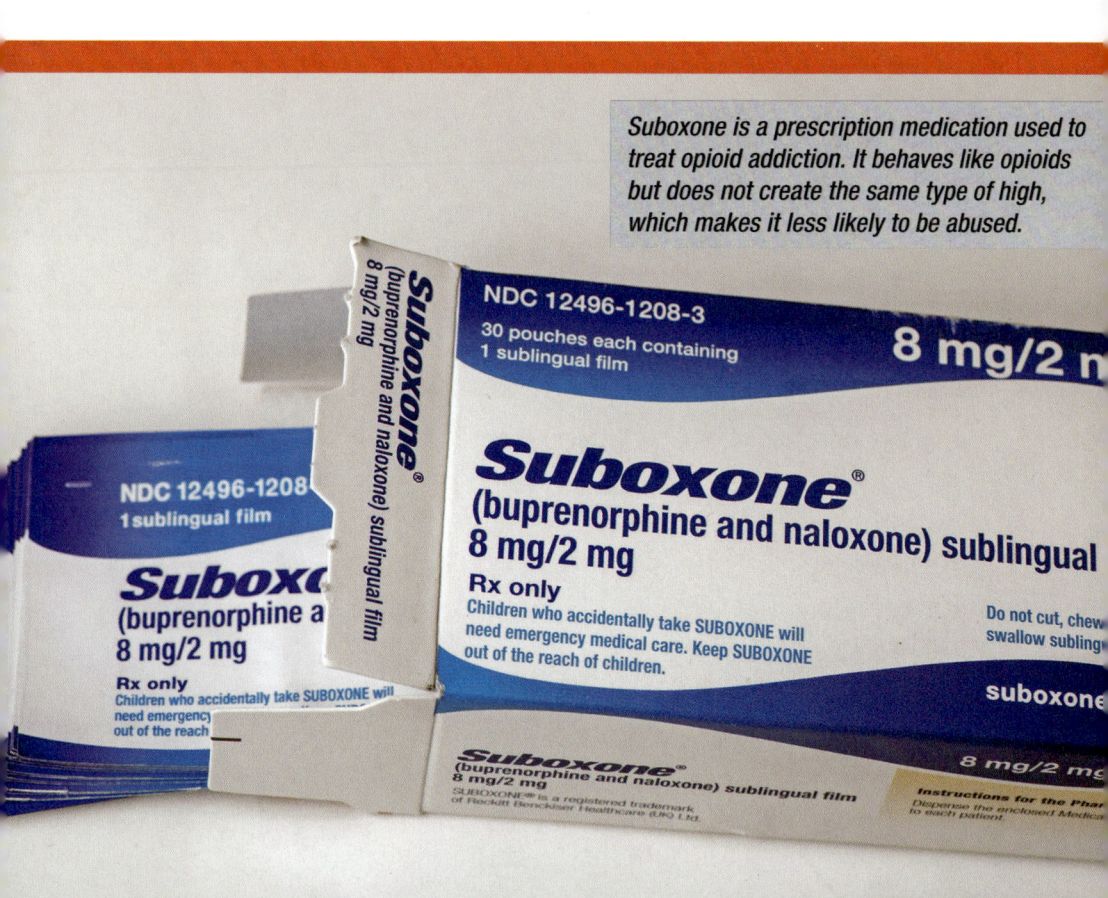

> "Treatment hasn't been readily available. It's difficult to get, expensive and not necessarily covered by insurance."[32]
>
> —Richard Schottenfeld, a professor of psychiatry at Yale School of Medicine

Suboxone is a prescription medication used to treat opioid addiction. It behaves like opioids but does not create the same type of high, which makes it less likely to be abused.

Online Addiction Support

Many people addicted to opioids want to get clean but lack access to resources to do so. The opioid epidemic has deeply impacted many rural communities, but treatment programs and support groups may be nonexistent or hard to come by in those areas. In some cases the nearest program may be many miles away.

Given the limited options, people are turning to online communities for recovery support. Numerous communities for people struggling with addiction exist on social platforms like Facebook and Reddit. These platforms connect people from around the country and offer a place to share their personal stories and support others with their own addiction struggles. The free cost, constant availability, and potential for anonymity make these groups appealing for some.

While medical professionals note the positive impact these communities can have, they worry the communities do not offer a complete recovery solution due to the unstructured format, lack of accountability, and the potential for misinformation to be circulated. Further, people offering advice may not have addiction training. Despite these concerns, Maggs Gibbons, who lives in a rural area of southern Illinois, where treatment options are very limited, finds online communities to be helpful in her recovery efforts: "I like being at home and having my phone on me and the support to help me, it means a lot. It's easier for me when I have a bad day to read someone else's story. Sometimes you need someone else to boost your confidence."

Quoted in Peter Allen Clark, "Getting Clean Online," Mashable, March 29, 2018. https://mashable.com.

Inpatient and Outpatient Treatment Programs

People who actively engage in inpatient and outpatient treatment programs boost their chances of overcoming addiction. Scientific research on recovery shows that the more focused someone is on recovery, the more likely he or she will maintain long-term sobriety, especially in the first eighteen months of recovery when the risk of relapse remains high.

Inpatient or residential treatment programs provide a place for program participants to live while they safely detox and learn tactics for managing and overcoming their addiction. These programs are typically staffed twenty-four hours a day with addiction specialists and last anywhere from 28 to 120 days. With residential treatment programs, drug users are removed from the people and environments that may encourage relapse. Program participants learn how to manage their symptoms and cravings within a structured setting at the rehab facility, with the aim of taking those skills back into their home environments as they reintegrate into routine life.

During treatment participants work with therapists to understand the underlying causes of their addiction. Getting clear about the people, issues, and environment that drive a desire to use drugs is key. Patients are taught to dismiss false beliefs and insecurities about themselves, given self-help tools to cope with their thoughts and emotions, and shown how to communicate more effectively. The ultimate goal is to give people the skills to avoid the triggers and cravings that caused them to rely on drugs in the past.

Participants also attend group sessions, in which they share their personal struggles of addiction among other people dealing with addiction. It can be helpful for people to realize they are not alone. Most programs also include a family therapy component, in which family members address family dynamics like codependency as well as feelings of anger and resentment. In some cases it is the first time family members have expressed their feelings openly with one another. Lastly, some treatment programs offer specialized sessions that teach additional coping techniques for handling stress, anger, and grief. Michelle, a participant at an inpatient treatment facility, describes the benefits of a long-term program: "The counseling I receive . . . is teaching me healthy coping mechanisms to deal with life's difficulties so I'll no longer want to use drugs. I am working to mend the relationships with my family and friends instead of dwelling on the mistakes of the past."[33]

> "I am working to mend the relationships with my family and friends instead of dwelling on the mistakes of the past."[33]
>
> —Michelle, a participant at an inpatient treatment facility

Those seeking help for opioid addiction may prefer outpatient treatment programs, which vary widely in terms of programming and required hours of attendance. These programs also offer therapy components but are less disruptive to a person's routine, since participants can continue to work or go to school. These programs tend to be more successful for those with a mild addiction versus a severe addiction.

Harm-Reduction Approaches

Harm-reduction strategies are a set of interventions that acknowledges the humanity of drug users. These strategies accept that both legal and illegal drug use is a part of society and will likely always be present in some shape or form. Rather than ignoring or punishing drug users, harm reduction works to reduce the harmful effects of drug use—with the aim of saving lives. It does so by providing care, services, and resources to minimize dangerous consequences of drug use. Two of the most effective strategies in reducing harm are needle exchange programs and the distribution of naloxone, an opioid overdose antidote that can completely reverse the effects of opioid overdose and prevent death.

Needle exchange programs are community-based programs that aim to reduce the spread of disease that can easily be transmitted through sharing needles. With many heroin users injecting as many as twelve times per day, they often reuse needles or share with other users. However, public health officials recommend that a clean needle be used for every injection. These programs give people sterile needles and syringes free of cost and a place to safely dispose of used needles and syringes. Program participants are encouraged to learn safe injection practices and wound care. Many of these exchanges also connect some of the hardest-to-reach people to other services and programs, including MAT programs, overdose prevention education, screening for transmitted diseases, vaccination for hepatitis A and B, and mental health services. Further, the collection of dirty needles promotes a safer environment for first responders and others in the community.

Critics of these programs believe they encourage illegal behavior. Brian Besser, an agent with the US Drug Enforcement Administration, says, "We're giving everything you need to be a heroin addict except for the heroin and the thumb that you need to push down on the plunger."[34] Despite such critics' opinions, in 2011 the US surgeon general determined that needle exchange programs reduce the risk of HIV and hepatitis among intravenous drug users, promote entry into treatment, and do not increase illegal drug use or crime.

Another harm-reduction strategy is naloxone distribution. Naloxone, commonly known by the brand name Narcan, is a nonaddictive medication that blocks the effects of opioids in the body—both the euphoria and the dangerous side effects. When a person overdoses, his or her breathing and heart rate typically slow, cutting off oxygen to the brain. Naloxone reverses respiratory depression by binding to the opioid receptors. It is administered via either a nasal spray or an intravenous injection into a muscle, into a vein, or under the skin. Usually within minutes of being administered, the naloxone helps a person breathe normally again. According to research from Brigham and Women's Hospital in Boston, naloxone reversed more than 93 percent of overdoses in which it was given to patients.

Given the rapid increase in overdoses in recent years, the US surgeon general issued an advisory in April 2018 recommending that more people carry naloxone. Many emergency medical personnel and other first responders carry it, but naloxone distribution programs also offer naloxone kits to opioid users, their families and friends, and other service providers who may witness an opioid overdose. According to the National Institute on Drug Abuse, from 1996 to 2014, laypersons reversed at least 26,500 opioid overdoses in the United States with naloxone. While naloxone is an important tool in saving overdose victims, it is not a long-term solution for opioid addiction: people still need to receive treatment.

Improving Pain Management

Some in the medical community believe that while opioids do serve a purpose, they are not an effective long-term solution for pain management. Instead, these professionals recommend that patients explore alternative treatments for pain. Some of these include over-the-counter pain relievers such as acetaminophen, aspirin, naproxen, and ibuprofen; nondrug remedies such as physical therapy, massage, yoga, and acupuncture; and high-tech

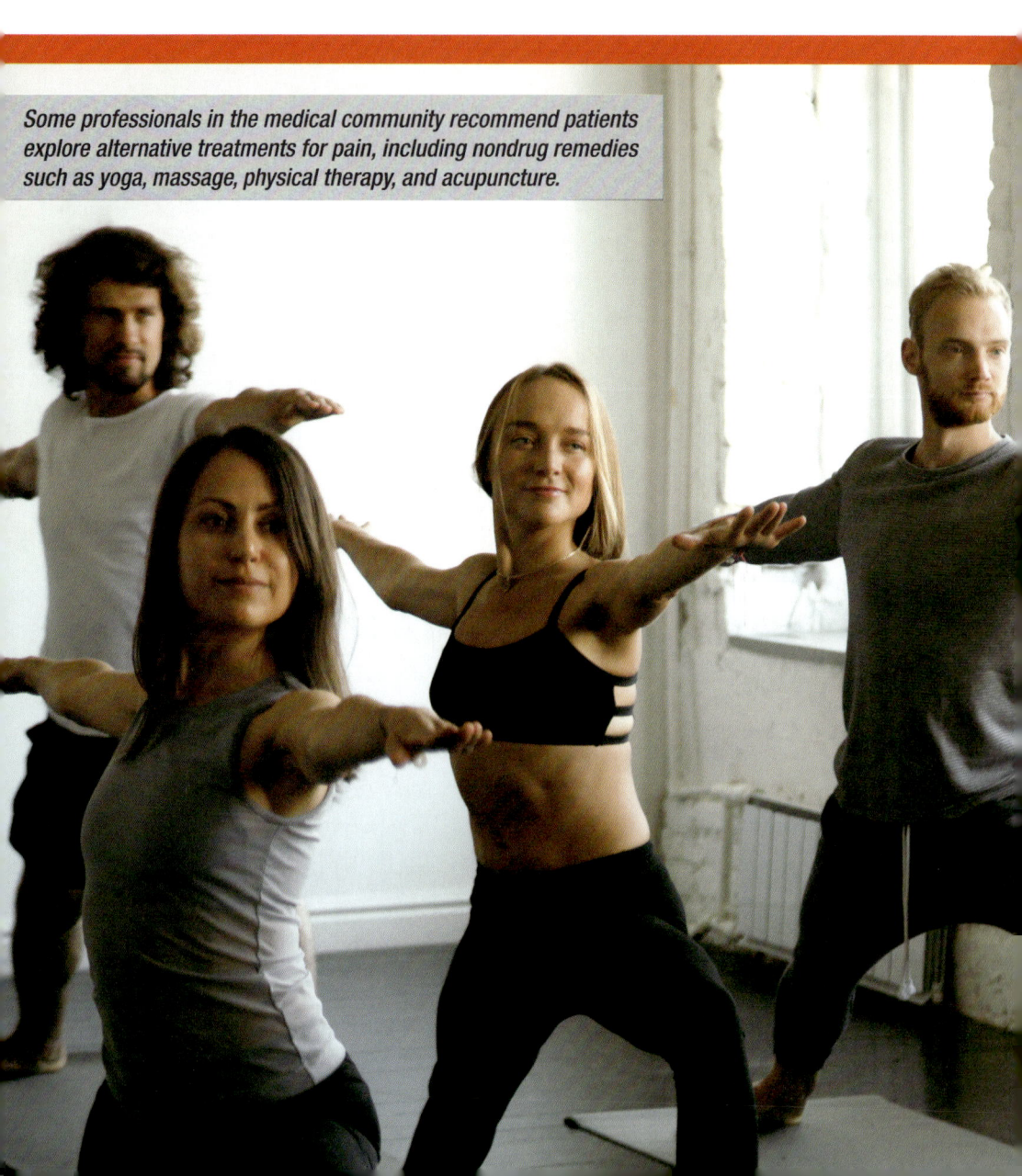

Some professionals in the medical community recommend patients explore alternative treatments for pain, including nondrug remedies such as yoga, massage, physical therapy, and acupuncture.

treatments that use electrical signals and radio waves to combat pain. One alternative being considered is marijuana, a drug derived from the cannabis plant. It can replace opioids as a pain reliever, ease withdrawal symptoms, and reduce the chances of relapse. Many consider it less addictive than other FDA-approved opioid replacement therapies and maintenance medications that can sometimes also be habit forming on their own.

While there is broad support in the medical community for alternative treatments, many obstacles limit people's access to them. In some cases, these types of treatments are not found in rural areas. Even if a doctor recommended an alternative treatment, a person might need to travel a significant distance to get to a treatment provider. In other cases, insurance companies either require prior authorizations before they cover treatment or require higher copays for services. If alternative treatments are not covered by insurance, they can be quite costly over time. Still, it is important that other options exist to reduce the number of people who take opioids in the first place—thus decreasing the number of people who become addicted.

While some strides have been made in treating opioid addiction, much more needs to be done to help save lives. Karen Boland, who lost her son to a heroin addiction in 2013, says, "We need doctors treating the mind and the addiction, which doesn't always happen. We need society to understand that addiction is a cycle of relapse and remission. We need society to understand that every addicted person is someone's child."[35]

Source Notes

Introduction: The Opioid Crisis: A Public Health Emergency

1. Quoted in Centers for Disease Control and Prevention, "Real Stories: Cortney," September 22, 2017. www.cdc.gov.
2. Quoted in US Department of Health and Human Services, "HHS Awards over $1 Billion to Combat the Opioid Crisis," September 19, 2018. www.hhs.gov.

Chapter One: The Scope of Opioid Addiction

3. Quoted in *Frontline*, "Heroin & Opioid Addiction, In Your Own Words: The Parent of an Addict from Payson, Ariz." http://apps.frontline.org.
4. Quoted in John Bacon, "'We Are Losing Too Many Americans': Suicides, Drug Overdoses Rise as US Life Expectancy Drops," *USA Today*, November 29, 2018. www.usatoday.com.
5. Quoted in *Frontline*, "Heroin & Opioid Addiction, In Your Own Words: Someone Who Treats Addiction in Asheville, N.C." http://apps.frontline.org.
6. Quoted in Tessie Castillo, "Should We Limit How Many Times Someone Is Saved with Naloxone?," Fix, November 15, 2016. www.thefix.com.

Chapter Two: What Influences Opioid Addiction?

7. Karen Boland, "A Mother's Guilt," *USA Today*, June 13, 2018. www.usatoday.com.
8. Elizabeth Brico, "My Trauma Led Me to Self-Medicate with Heroin," *Tonic* (blog), *Vice*, January 30, 2018. https://tonic.vice.com.
9. Quoted in Brico, "My Trauma Led Me to Self-Medicate with Heroin."
10. Quoted in Elsevier, "GWAS Identifies Genetic Alteration Associated with Opioid Dependence," February 22, 2018. www.elsevier.com.

Chapter Three: How People Become Addicted to Opioids

11. Quoted in *Vice*, "Fentanyl: The Drug Deadlier than Heroin," YouTube, July 22, 2016. www.youtube.com.
12. Quoted in Stay Safe Oregon, "Real Stories: Randi's Story," 2019. https://staysafeoregon.com.
13. Rocco Merolli, "What Is It like to Withdraw from Opioids?," Quora, September 23, 2015. www.quora.com.
14. Maia Szalavitz, *Unbroken Brain: A Revolutionary New Way of Understanding Addiction*. New York: Picador, 2016, p. 33.
15. Quoted in Ruben Castaneda, "Why Some Opioids Users Don't Fear a Fatal Overdose," *U.S. News & World Report*, April 23, 2018. https://health.usnews.com.
16. Quoted in Sarah T. Williams, "What's It Really like to Withdraw from Heroin and Painkillers?," MinnPost, February 14, 2014. www.minnpost.com.
17. Quoted in Shreeya Sinha, "A Visual Journey Through Addiction," *New York Times*, December 18, 2018. www.nytimes.com.

Chapter Four: Living with Opioid Addiction

18. Quoted in Rene Wisely, "Why Are Hep C Infections Skyrocketing? Opioid Abuse to Blame," *Wellness & Prevention* (blog), Michigan Health, January 2, 2018. https://healthblog.uofmhealth.org.
19. Quoted in Abby Goodnough, "Costly to Treat, Hepatitis C Gains Quietly in U.S.," *New York Times*, July 23, 2015. www.nytimes.com.
20. Quoted in *Vice*, "Fentanyl."
21. Niko McManus, "The Effects of Isolation on Addiction," AddictionCenter, March 23, 2016. www.addictioncenter.com.
22. Susana Ferreira, "Portugal's Radical Drugs Policy Is Working. Why Hasn't the World Copied It?," *Guardian* (Manchester), December 5, 2017. www.theguardian.com.
23. Quoted in Sinha, "A Visual Journey Through Addiction."

24. Quoted in Yuki Noguchi, "Anguished Families Shoulder the Biggest Burdens of Opioid Addiction," NPR, April 18, 2018. www.npr.org.
25. Quoted in Noguchi, "Anguished Families Shoulder the Biggest Burdens of Opioid Addiction."
26. Quoted in NPR, "We Found Joy: An Addict Struggles to Get Treatment," May 5, 2016. www.npr.org.

Chapter Five: Overcoming Opioid Addiction

27. Quoted in Tracey Duncan, "Quitting Opioids Cold Turkey Made Me Want to Die," *Tonic* (blog), *Vice*, November 27, 2017. https://tonic.vice.com.
28. Quoted in Williams, "What's It Really like to Withdraw from Heroin and Painkillers?"
29. Quoted in Kathy Jean Schultz, "A Former Opioid Addict at Harvard Says We're Getting Addiction Wrong," Daily Beast, November 27, 2018. www.thedailybeast.com.
30. Quoted in BAART Programs, "'Focus on Your Recovery!' A Methadone Treatment Success Story," August 8, 2017. https://baartprograms.com.
31. Quoted in Workit Health, "From Heroin User to Health Advocate: Suboxone Success Story," January 30, 2018. www.workithealth.com.
32. Quoted in Yale Medicine, "Overcoming Opioid Addiction: A Woman Shares Her Story," February 27, 2018. www.yalemedicine.org.
33. AppleGate Recovery, "Michelle's Story: It Can Happen to Anyone." https://applegaterecovery.com.
34. Quoted in Matthew Piper, "Critics Say Syringe Exchange 'Party Packs' Enable Drug Use and Add Needles to the Streets, While Providers Say They're Saving Lives," *Salt Lake (UT) Tribune*, August 5, 2017. www.sltrib.com.
35. Boland, "A Mother's Guilt."

Get Help and Information

Behavioral Health Treatment Services Locator
Substance Abuse and Mental Health Services Administration (SAMHSA)
5600 Fishers Ln.
Rockville, MD 20857
website: https://findtreatment.samhsa.gov

SAMHSA's online resource locator allows users to search for mental health and substance abuse treatment facilities located throughout the United States, including physicians and programs offering methadone and buprenorphine treatment. The website also includes links to a national helpline and several addiction self-help and peer-support groups.

Faces of Opioids
website: www.facebook.com/groups/facesofopioids

Now a nonprofit opioid awareness organization, the Faces of Opioids began as a Facebook group for people struggling with or impacted by opioid addiction. Participants share personal stories and photos in an effort not only to show the prevalence of addiction but also to shift the stigma associated with it. The group is intended to be a safe space for people to connect with and offer support for one another.

Harm Reduction Coalition
22 W. Twenty-Seventh St., Fifth Floor
New York, NY 10001
website: https://harmreduction.org

The Harm Reduction Coalition advocates for individuals and communities impacted by drug use and strives to promote the rights of and social inclusion for drug users. Its website offers a variety of tools and methods for reducing the harm related to drug use. Informative resources include brochures, fact sheets, training programs, videos, and podcasts.

National Institute on Drug Abuse (NIDA)
6001 Executive Blvd.
Rockville, MD 20852
website: www.drugabuse.gov

The NIDA is a federal research institute that uses science to better understand drug abuse and addiction. Its website provides a whole section devoted to opioids, with informational pages, research reports, videos, research findings, and various publications on opioids. It also includes a link to the NIDA publication "Opioid Facts for Teens," which provides facts about opioids in a question-and-answer format.

National Opioid Crisis
US Department of Health and Human Services (HHS)
200 Independence Ave. SW
Washington, DC 20201
website: www.hhs.gov

This HHS website is dedicated solely to providing help, resources, and information about the national opioid crisis, prevention, treatment, and recovery. It includes discussion of the HHS's five-point strategy to combat the opioid crisis, which includes better prevention, treatment, and recovery services; better data; better pain management; better targeting of overdose reversal drugs; and better research.

Opioid Watch
website: https://opioidinstitute.org

An independent, nonprofit website, Opioid Watch offers original news and commentary on the opioid crisis to those seeking solutions, including public health officials, physicians, and patients.

Along with research topics such as addiction, chronic pain, fentanyl, and treatment, the website provides basic information about opioids and the latest opioid overdose statistics.

Partnership for Drug-Free Kids + Center on Addiction
633 Third Ave., Nineteenth Floor
New York, NY 10011
website: https://drugfree.org

Partnership for Drug-Free Kids is a national nonprofit organization dedicated to supporting families of addicted individuals. Its website offers access to the Medicine Abuse Project, a campaign to end medicine abuse; an Opioid Crisis portal for resources to understand and take steps to address the current epidemic; and specialists trained to help families develop personalized action plans for addressing opioid abuse.

For Further Research

Books

Nonfiction

Maureen Cavanagh, *If You Love Me: A Mother's Journey Through Her Daughter's Opioid Addiction*. New York: Holt, 2018.

Ryan Hampton, *American Fix: Inside the Opioid Addiction Crisis—and How to End It*. New York: All Points, 2018.

Beth Macy, *Dopesick: Dealers, Doctors, and the Drug Company That Addicted America*. New York: Little, Brown, 2018.

John Perritano, *Opioids: Heroin, OxyContin, and Painkillers*. Broomall, PA: Mason Crest, 2016.

Sam Quinones, *Dreamland (YA Edition): The True Tale of America's Opiate Epidemic*. New York: Bloomsbury YA, 2019.

Maia Szalavitz, *Unbroken Brain: A Revolutionary New Way of Understanding Addiction*. New York: Picador, 2016.

Fiction

Mindy McGinnis, *Heroine*. New York: Tegan, 2019.

Nico Walker, *Cherry: A Novel*. New York: Knopf, 2018.

Internet Sources

American Society of Addiction Medicine, "Opioid Addiction Treatment: A Guide for Patients, Family and Friends," 2016. http://eguideline.guidelinecentral.com.

CNN, "Opioid Crisis Fast Facts," January 16, 2019. www.cnn.com.

Frontline, "Heroin & Opioid Addiction, In Your Own Words." http://apps.frontline.org.

Jennifer Harlan, "'You Can Make It Out': Readers Share Stories of Opioid Addiction and Survival," *New York Times*, December 27, 2018. www.nytimes.com.

Peter Jamison, "Falling Out," *Washington Post*, December 18, 2018. www.washingtonpost.com.

National Institute on Drug Abuse, "Opioid Facts for Teens," July 10, 2018. www.drugabuse.gov.

Shreeya Sinha, "A Visual Journey Through Addiction," *New York Times*, December 18, 2018. www.nytimes.com.

Vice, "Fentanyl: The Drug Deadlier than Heroin," YouTube, July 22, 2016. www.youtube.com.

Laura Wamsley, "Fentanyl Surpasses Heroin as Drug Most Often Involved in Deadly Overdoses," NPR, December 12, 2018. www.npr.org.

Index

Note: Boldface page numbers indicate illustrations.

abstinence-based treatment programs, 54–55
addiction
  as behavioral choice, 20
  as disease of brain, 9, 20
  method of consumption of drugs and, 22, **24**
  as process taking place over time, 34
  See also opioid addiction
addictive personality myth, 26
adolescents
  drug use and family situation of, 20–21
  risk factors for drug use, 21–22
  vulnerability to addiction, 16–17
African Americans and addiction, 14–15
alcohol consumption and drug addiction, 21
Altarum, 50–51
anxiety, 29
attachment theory, 29
Azar, Alex, 8

Behavioral Health Treatment Services Locator, Substance Abuse and Mental Health Services Administration (SAMHSA), 67
behavioral risk factors, 22, **23**
Benton, Sherry, 52
Besser, Brian, 61
Boland, Karen, 25, 63
brain
  addiction as disease of, 9, 20
  changes in chemistry of, 33–34
  circuits and variant near RGMA gene, 28–29
  dopamine and, 33, **35**
  neuroimaging of, 38
  opioid use and development of, 17
  rewiring of circuits, 33–34
  stimulation of reward center, 32–33
Brico, Elizabeth, 18, 26–27
Brigham and Women's Hospital (Boston), 61
buprenorphine, 56

Centers for Disease Control
and Prevention (CDC)
  on adolescents and
    addiction, 16–17
  correlation of increase in
    opioid prescriptions to
    overdose deaths, 6
  deaths from opioids (1999–
    2017), 5
  increase in hepatitis C as
    result of increased opioid
    use, 42–43
  nonfatal overdoses (2016–
    2017), 19
  on opioid prescriptions, 31
  race and opioid-related
    deaths, 14–15
"chasing the dragon," 34
chronic conditions, 6
chronic pain
  as disease, 31
  number of Americans
    experiencing, 30
  opioid receptors and, 32
  opioids prescribed to
    alleviate, 31
Civil War, 13
comorbidity, described, 23
costs of opioid addiction,
  48–51

deaths from overdoses
  addict's awareness of
    possibility of, 37–38
  effects on families, 47–48
  from fentanyl
    in 2017, 17
    from 1999 to 2017, **16**
    of African Americans, 15
    versus heroin (2016), 7
    testing strips and, 56
  from heroin, 7, **16**
  in New York City (2016), 47
  from opioids
    in 2017, 9
    from 1999 to 2017, 5, 6,
      16
    of African Americans,
      14–15
    correlation of increase in
      opioid prescriptions to, 6
    daily, 17
    of famous individuals, 14,
      15, 19
    states with highest, 12
  from prescription painkillers,
    16
  relapse and, 55
dependence, 34
depression, 23–25, 38–39
detoxification programs,
  52–53, **54**
dopamine, 33, **35**
drug rehab. *See* treatment

emotional effects of opioid
  addiction, 43–46, **44**
environmental risk factors,
  20–22, **23**, 28
epidemic, beginning of, 5–7

Faces of Opioids (website), 67
families
  dysfunctional, and drug use, 21, 46
  effects of opioid addiction on, 46–48
  therapy and, 59
fentanyl, **6**
  allure of, 18
  cost of, 48
  deaths
    in 2017, 17
    from 1999 to 2017, **16**
    of African Americans and, 15
    versus heroin deaths (2016), 7
    testing strips and, 56
  illicit version of, 7
  mixed with heroin, 12
  potency of, 7, 17
  symptoms of overdose, 40–41
  testing strips, 56
  unknowing consumption of, 18–19
  withdrawal, 18
Ferreira, Susana, 45–46
fight/flight response, 27
financial effects of opioid addiction, 48–51
Fontana, Robert, 43
foster care system, growth of, 50

friends, effects of opioid addiction on, 46–48

Gelernter, Joel, 29
gender and use of opioids, 15–16
genetics and risk of addiction, 28–29
Gibbons, Maggs, 58
Grahovac, Ivana, 39

Harm Reduction Coalition, 67–68
harm-reduction strategies, 60–61
Harrison Narcotics Tax Act (1914), 13
hepatitis C, 42–43, 61
heroin
  additives in, 41
  "chasing the dragon" and, 34
  increase in use and deaths, 7, **16**
  methadone and, 55
  for pain management, 13
  as substitute for opioids, 7
  types of, 12
  use in US, 12

inpatient treatment programs, 58–59
isolation and addiction, **44**, 44–45

Johnson, Destini, 49

lawsuits, 47

marijuana, 63
marketing, 47
McCandless, Mandy, 46
McMahon, Michael E., 47
McManus, Niko, 45
medication-assisted treatment (MAT), 55–57, **57**
mental illness, as risk factor, 23–25
Merolli, Rocco, 36
methadone, 55
morphine, 5, 13, 27
Myer, Marc, 39
myth of addictive personality, 26

naloxone (Narcan), 19, 56, 60, 61
National Center for PTSD, 26–27
National Institute on Drug Abuse (NIDA)
  about, 68
  genetics and risk for addiction, 28
  neuroimaging of brain, 38
  number of fentanyl drug overdose deaths (2017), 17
  number of layperson-reversed opioid overdoses (1996–2014), 61
National Institutes of Health, 12, 38
National Opioids Crisis (website), 68
National Survey on Drug Use and Health (2016), 12
needle exchange programs, 60–61
New York City, 47

online recovery support, 58
opioid addiction
  as accidental, 10
  as chronic disease, 9, 20, 40
  consequences of, 17–19
  effects on
    family and friends, 46–48
    financial, 48–51
    physical, 40–43, **42**
    psychological and emotional, 43–46, **44**
  as global problem, 11–12
  lowering of inhibitions, 43
  number of Americans suffering from (2016), 12
  number of Americans suffering from (2017), 4
  signs of, 10–11
  transmission of other diseases and, 42–43

opioid manufacturers, lawsuit against, 47
opioids
  most popular prescribed, 13
  naturally produced by body, 33
  types of, 5, 12
opioid use disorder, 9
  See also opioid addiction
Opioid Watch (website), 68–69
opium, history of use in US, 13
outpatient treatment programs, 60
overdoses
  allure of risk of, 18
  cost of emergency care for, 50
  naloxone to reverse, 19, 60, 61
  number of nonfatal, 19
  symptoms of, 40–41
  See also deaths from overdoses

Page, Mike, 19
pain management
  alternative treatments for, **62**, 62–63
  heroin for, 13
  morphine for, 13
  opioids prescribed for, 5–7, **6**
Partnership for Drug-Free Kids + Center on Addiction, 69
peer pressure, 21
Petty, Tom, **15**
Philadelphia, 13
physical effects of opioid addiction, 40–43, **42**
post-traumatic stress disorder (PTSD) as risk factor, 25–28, **27**
prescription opioids, 31–32
Prince, 19
psychological effects of opioid addiction, 43–46, **44**
psychological risk factors, 23–25

race and use of opioids, 14–15
relapse
  abstinence-based treatment programs and, 54–55
  death and, 55
  foster care and, 50
  gender and, 16
  rates, 38
  reasons for, 38–39
  time of highest risk of, 58
residential treatment programs, 58–59
RGMA gene, variant near, 28–29

risk factors for addiction
  environmental and social, 20–22, **23**, 28
  genetics, 28–29
  psychological conditions, 23–25
  trauma and PTSD, 25–28, **27**
Roiphe, Emily Carter, 53
RTI International, 56

Saint Louis University, 24
Schottenfeld, Richard, 57
Schuchat, Anne, 14
Searp, Jerry, 43
self-hatred, 44
Sexton, Dale, 47–48
Sexton, Katy, 47–48
Sexton, Melissa, 47–48
sexual abuse, as cause of PTSD, 27
social media, recovery support on, 58
social risk factors, 20–22
Suboxone, 56, **57**
Substance Abuse and Mental Health Services Administration, 4
Szalavitz, Maia, 26, 36

teenagers
  drug use and family situation of, 20–21
  risk factors for drug use, 21–22

vulnerability to addiction, 16–17
tolerance, 33, 34
trauma as risk factor, 25–28, **27**
treatment
  abstinence-based programs, 54–55
  cost of, 48–49
  detoxification programs, 52–53, **54**
  grants from HHS, 8
  importance of supportive setting for, 53, **54**
  inpatient (residential) programs, 58–59
  medication-assisted programs, 55–57, **57**
  obstacles to getting, 57, 63
  online recovery support, 58
  social media and, 58
Turner, Wendi, 50

Unbroken Brain: A Revolutionary New Way of Understanding Addiction (Szalavitz), 26
US Department of Health and Human Services (HHS)
  grants to fight opioid crisis, 8
  increase in foster care population, 50

National Opioids Crisis
   website, 68
number addicted to opioids,
   12
users
   locations of, 12, 13
   number of, 12
US Food and Drug
   Administration (FDA), 13

van der Kolk, Bessel, 27

Volkow, Nora, 54–55

Wakhlu, Sidarth, 37–38
war, as cause of PTSD, 27, **27**
withdrawal, **37**
   from fentanyl, 18
   medications and, 55
   symptoms of, 35–36
World Health Organization,
   7–8

Picture Credits

Cover: Juanmonino/iStockphoto.com

6: PureRadiancePhoto/Shutterstock.com
10: Marjan Apostolovic/Shutterstock.com
15: Jack Fordyce/Shutterstock.com
16: Maury Aaseng
23: Lopolo/Shutterstock.com
24: Ttatty/Shutterstock.com
27: BPTU/Shutterstock.com
32: sirtravelalot/Shutterstock.com
35: Andrii Vodolazhskyi/Shutterstock.com
37: Izf/Shutterstock.com
42: sciencepics/Shutterstock.com
44: Sam Wordley/Shuttestock.com
49: Monkey Business Images/Shutterstock.com
54: Rapeepat Pornsipak/Shutterstock.com
57: katz/Shutterstock.com
62: fizkes/Shutterstock.com

About the Author

Jennifer Skancke is a freelance editor and writer living in Seattle, Washington.